THE 30-DAY LOW-CARB DIET SOLUTION

Michael R. Eades, M.D.

Mary Dan Eades, M.D.

WILEY

John Wiley & Sons, Inc.

Published by John Wiley & Sons, Inc., Hoboken, New Jersey
Published simultaneously in Canada

Design and production by Navta Associates, Inc.

Limit of Liability/Disclaimer of Warranty: While the publisher and the author have used their best efforts in preparing this book, they make no representations or warranties with respect to the accuracy or completeness of the contents of this book and specifically disclaim any implied warranties of merchantability or fitness for a particular purpose. No warranty may be created or extended by sales representatives or written sales materials. The advice and strategies contained herein may not be suitable for your situation. You should consult with a professional where appropriate. Neither the publisher nor the author shall be liable for any loss of profit or any other commercial damages, including but not limited to special, incidental, consequential, or other damages.

For general information about our other products and services, please contact our Customer Care Department within the United States at (800) 762-2974, outside the United States at (317) 572-3993 or fax (317) 572-4002.

Wiley also publishes its books in a variety of electronic formats. Some content that appears in print may not be available in electronic books.

Library of Congress Cataloging-in-Publication Data:
Eades, Michael R.
  The 30-day low-carb diet solution / Michael R. Eades, Mary Dan Eades.
      p. ; cm.
Includes bibliographical references and index.
  ISBN 0-471-43050-1 (cloth : alk. paper)
  ISBN 0-471-45415-X (paper)
  1. Low-carbohydrate diet. 2. Low-carbohydrate diet—Recipes.
  [DNLM: 1. Diet, Reducing—Popular Works. 2. Dietary Carbohydrates—administration & dosage—Popular Works. WD 212 E11z 2003] I. Title: Thirty-day low-carb diet solution. II. Eades, Mary Dan. III. Title.
  RM237.73 .E227 2003
  613.2'83—dc21

                          2002014905

Printed in the United States of America

10 9 8 7 6 5 4 3 2 1

We dedicate this book to our grandsons,
Thomas Michael Eades
and William Alexander Eades,
Who make life worthwhile.

Contents

Acknowledgments v

Introduction 1

CHAPTER 1 Why Low-Carb Works 3

CHAPTER 2 Getting Ready to Go Low-Carb 24

CHAPTER 3 So . . . What Do I Eat? 33

CHAPTER 4 The 30-Day Low-Carb Diet Solution
Meal Plans 44

CHAPTER 5 Recipes 71

APPENDIX A Carbohydrate Content of Combination Foods
(Dairy, Nuts, Soy) 169

Resources 171

Meal Planner Worksheet 172

APPENDIX B Recommended Multivitamin
and Mineral Profile 173

APPENDIX C Visualizing Meat Portion Sizes 174

APPENDIX D Protein Requirements 176

Index 178

Acknowledgments

Although this book, like our previous ones, is an outgrowth of our nearly twenty years of experience in using low-carb nutrition to help patients and readers control their weight and weight-related health problems, it's a great departure in its simplicity. For that we owe a debt of gratitude to Gary Taubes for his *New York Times Sunday Magazine* cover story that vindicated low-carb dieting in the minds of almost all its critics. Thanks to that piece, we were able to do something we had wanted to do since 1995—write a low-carb book devoid of heavy scientific explanations and complex formulae, one that would just tell folks what to eat.

Of course, the book would never have found its congenial home without the tireless efforts of our ever-faithful agents, Channa Taub and Carol Mann.

And a big thanks to our editor Tom Miller and the many people at John Wiley & Sons, who not only enthusiastically embraced the notion of our writing a really simple low-carb primer, but collectively exerted Herculean effort to bring it out in record time.

A special thanks to our partners at Advanced Metabolics, Larry McCleary, MD, Christine McCleary, and Brett Astor, who struggled to work around the havoc that this expedited project caused as well as for listening to us whine about it.

To Rose Crane, many thanks for developing many of the recipes; it made the job infinitely easier.

No project we undertake would ever come to pass without the help of our loyal and friendly staff. A big thanks to our nurse Debbie Judd and our executive assistant Kristi McAfee who toil away on our behalf at all hours of the night and day. We really do notice, guys, and appreciate it more than you know.

And finally, thanks and love to our wonderful family—sons Ted, Dan, and Scott, daughters-in-law, Jamye and Katherine, and the joys of our life, our grandsons, Thomas and William—for whom we always do everything we do.

Introduction

We've been powering the low-carbohydrate movement since the mid-1980s, when we first began using carb restriction to effectively treat our patients who suffered from high blood pressure, heart disease, diabetes, overweight, and a host of other medical ills related to disordered metabolism. In 1989, in *Thin So Fast,* we described, for the first time for the layman, the theory of a connection between all these diseases and the hormone insulin. (At the time, the connection was speculative; now it's all been borne out in the research lab.)

Five or six years later, having dug out and assembled a wealth of medical research supporting this theory, we were able to lay out all the science behind why a protein-rich low-carbohydrate diet accomplishes what a low-fat diet can't in our 1996 book, *Protein Power.* The international scientific research continued apace, and in 2000 we streamlined and updated the nutritional information and expanded the program into a comprehensive lifestyle for good health in *The Protein Power LifePlan,* again laying out all the scientific underpinnings in support of our program.

We felt that taking a position that ran counter to the prevailing medical "wisdom" demanded a full display of the scientific rationale behind it, not only to give our readers added comfort in adopting this diet and lifestyle, but to silence the critics—a job that proved to be a tough uphill battle against the entrenched forces of the high-carb/low-fat devoted. But what reams of scientific papers had been unable to do, a journalist's pen accomplished. Now, the protein-rich, low-carb diet has arrived, finally having been vindicated on the July 7, 2002 cover of the Sunday Magazine of the venerable *New York Times Magazine,* in Gary Taubes' insightful article, *What if Fat Doesn't Make You Fat?* Suddenly the tide has turned.

Now, legions of overweight people who have struggled (and often failed) to keep their cholesterol, blood pressure, and blood sugar under control following the standard low-fat dietary prescription are standing on the platform, eager to board the low-carb train—all they want to know is how to do it. And so, we came to write *The 30-Day Low-Carb Diet Solution.*

Unlike any of our previous books on the subject—or, for that matter, any of the familiar books on low-carbing, such as *Enter the Zone, Dr. Atkins' Diet Revolution, Sugar Busters!, The Carbohydrate Addict's Diet,* or *The Paleo Diet*—in this book you'll find little or no science. There are no complicated charts or tables to use, no complex system of food combining, only the briefest of sketches of what a low-carb diet is and why it works; the balance of the book is simply how-to—how to easily determine how much protein and how much carb are right for you and how to go about eating it. If you do want to know all the science behind low-carb—every why, what, and how—pick up a copy of *Protein Power* and *The Protein Power LifePlan,* where you'll find the full story.

If you're now convinced of the merits of cutting carbs, don't give a flip about the science, and just want somebody to tell you what to eat, this is the book for you. In *The 30-Day Low-Carb Diet Solution,* you'll find ultra-simple guidelines that will let you get started on your low-carb journey today, plus dozens of easy and quick low-carb recipes, and even 30 days of low-carb meal plans to take all the guesswork out of eating. Once you're hooked on the low-carb way, you'll also want to pick up a copy of our new *Low-Carb Comfort Food Cookbook,* where you'll find hundreds of ways to indulge your passions for foods you never thought could be low-carb: fried chicken, breads and muffins warm from the oven, pizza, pasta, pies, cakes, and many more. Keeping your commitment to low-carb eating will be easier than ever before. So enjoy great eating—and lose weight while you're doing it.

CHAPTER 1

Why Low-Carb Works

If you're among the millions of people who have cut dietary fat to the bone in an attempt to lose weight, reduce cholesterol or triglycerides, or lower blood pressure only to have your efforts rewarded with frustration and failure, you're not alone. If you've done everything you were told to do by carefully following a low-fat, high-carbohydrate diet, struggling to try to reclaim your health and fitness, and failed—stop blaming yourself! You didn't fail at your diet—your diet failed you.

Victims of the Low-Fat Lie

As a society, North Americans responded to the constant urging of the media—television, newspapers, magazines, and talk shows—to reduce dietary fat, cutting our fat intake by almost 30 percent over the past two decades or so, and yet more of us are fatter today than ever before. If dietary fat had been the culprit behind the many diseases blamed on it, we'd be a nation of thin, healthy people by now. But, of course, we aren't.

In the fifteen to twenty years we've been trimming the fat, type II diabetes has tripled and in the last decade alone, obesity has increased by 30 percent. And now deaths from stroke and heart disease are on the rise. Far from solving the health problems that bedevil North Americans, eating more carbs and less fat made them substantially worse. And now the truth has finally come out: fat was never the problem. Elevated insulin, caused by the force-feeding of low-fat and no-fat carbs, has been responsible for causing so many of us to become overweight and develop high blood pressure as well as elevated blood sugar, cholesterol, and triglycerides.

Have you been on the wrong diet? Take this quiz and see.

	Yes	No
1. Have you gained weight on a low-fat diet?	☐	☐
2. While following a low-fat diet did your cholesterol rise?	☐	☐
3. While following a low-fat diet did your triglycerides rise?	☐	☐
4. Did you develop fluid retention or high blood pressure?	☐	☐
5. If female, during pregnancy did you develop gestational diabetes or toxemia?	☐	☐
6. Do you suffer an energy slump in the middle of the morning following a low-fat, high-carbohydrate breakfast or in mid-afternoon after a carb-rich lunch?	☐	☐
7. Do you tend to gain weight around your mid-section?	☐	☐
8. Do you suffer from acid reflux?	☐	☐
9. Do you suffer from gout?	☐	☐
10. Do you snore loudly and thrash the bedcovers when you sleep?	☐	☐

If you've answered "yes" to any of these questions, the low-fat diet has been the wrong diet for you; you'll reclaim your health and lose excess weight much more easily by switching to the low-carbohydrate diet. Let's take a quick look at why. (If you're already convinced and ready to go low-carb and want to skip even this brief explanatory background material, turn to Chapter 2.)

Before you read the following information, test your current nutritional knowledge.

Are the following statements true or false?

	True	False
1. Humans can survive and thrive without eating any carbohydrates whatsoever.	☐	☐
2. Eating a potato is like eating a quarter of a cup of pure sugar.	☐	☐
3. Good sources of protein are meat, fish, poultry, and eggs.	☐	☐
4. Anything made of wheat or corn—including pasta, bread, crackers, bagels, and chips—causes a rise in blood sugar and insulin.	☐	☐
5. The total carbohydrate of a food is the sum of the sugars, starches, and fiber it contains.	☐	☐
6. Eating protein causes a modest balanced rise in both insulin and glucagon.	☐	☐
7. The diet the USDA recommends—as shown in the USDA Food Pyramid—is almost identical to the balance of nutrients farmers use to fatten cattle and hogs on the feed lot.	☐	☐
8. Fat has virtually no effect on blood sugar, insulin, or glucagon.	☐	☐
9. As many as three out of four North Americans have a tendency to overproduce insulin when they eat starch or sugar.	☐	☐

                                                    True   False

10. Three out of four North Americans are
    overweight to some degree.   ☐   ☐

(Answers on page 23.)

The Metabolic Balance Scale

The body likes to keep its blood sugar within a fairly narrow "comfort" zone, neither too high nor too low. Throughout the day, blood sugar rises and falls outside this zone many times, but when it does the body normally marshals the hormonal forces necessary to restore it to a comfortable balance right away. For instance, when your blood sugar rises after a starchy meal or a sugary beverage, insulin—as the hormone chiefly responsible for regulating carbohydrate metabolism—acts quickly to bring it back down, by driving the sugar from the blood and into the cells where it can be burned for energy or stored for later use. When blood sugar dips too low, as it may overnight or if you go too long without eating, the body releases glucagon—insulin's partner hormone—to bring it back up into balance.

Tipping the Scale

Unfortunately, as medical studies have shown, about three out of four North Americans produce too much insulin when they eat a diet high in carbohydrates (grains, starchy vegetables, and sugars)—the very prescription laid out as dietary gospel in the low-fat, high-carb food pyramid. And when they do, their metabolic balance tips to the side of hyperinsulinemia (too much insulin in the blood), which is very likely the reason that a recent Harris poll indicates that three out of four North Americans are overweight to some degree.

You can think of insulin (and all hormones) as chemical messengers capable of "talking" to various tissues throughout the body that have built-in receivers to pick up the message. The receivers for insulin's message (called insulin receptors) lie on the surfaces of the muscle, liver, and fat cells, as well as certain cells in the kidney and in the appetite control centers of the brain. If the system is working normally, a rise in blood sugar signals the body to release insulin, which sends its message throughout the body to activate the insulin receptors, which in turn cause the sugar to leave the blood and move into the cells, returning the blood sugar to the comfort zone.

In many people, however, this system doesn't work normally. These people experience an exaggerated release of insulin when their blood sugar rises, and this excess begins to dull the response of the insulin receptors—over time, a condition called insulin resistance results. Once this occurs, insulin's message becomes so muted that the receivers can't hear it anymore and respond. Despite an excess of insulin in the blood, the blood sugar remains elevated. To overcome the resistance, the body then must shout louder by releasing even more insulin for its blood-sugar-lowering message to be heard. And a vicious cycle ensues of requiring ever-higher amounts of insulin to get the blood sugar back into balance; for many, diabetes ultimately results.

Unfortunately, regulating blood sugar is only one of insulin's many metabolic jobs and when it has accomplished the task of restoring blood sugar to normal, the excess is free to roam throughout the body, talking to other tissues, transmitting other messages. For instance, insulin tells the kidneys to hold on to salt (sodium). Where salt goes fluid follows, and the result is fluid retention. Insulin causes an increase in the thickness and constriction of artery walls as well; coupled with fluid retention, constriction of arteries can lead to high blood pressure. In the liver, insulin's message stimulates the production of excess cholesterol and triglycerides. Insulin tells the fat cells to store incoming calories as fat and keep them there—the fat cells become resistant to giving up their stored calories to burn for energy when insulin levels are high. And finally, in the muscles, which rely on burning fat as their preferred fuel source, insulin blocks the effective burning of fat for energy.

If three-quarters of us put out too much insulin when we eat carbohydrates, it's easy to see how following the low-fat, high-carb diet would have landed us exactly where it did—overweight, out of shape, and at greater risk for heart disease, diabetes, high blood pressure, gout, sleep apnea, and more. If excess insulin is the problem, then reducing insulin must be the answer. How do we reduce it? By diet and diet alone. All the major drug companies are spending billions of dollars searching for a drug that will lower insulin levels, but as of yet, all have failed in their quest. Currently, a common-sense, low-carbohydrate diet is the only viable way to rapidly and successfully lower insulin levels and begin to undo the damage caused by insulin resistance and hyperinsulinemia.

How can you tell if you're at risk for developing any insulin-related health problems? Complete the following personal health inventory.

	Yes	No
1. Do you have adult onset diabetes?	☐	☐
2. Did you develop diabetes during pregnancy?	☐	☐
3. Do you have elevated triglycerides?	☐	☐
4. Is your "good" HDL cholesterol level low?	☐	☐
5. Are you overweight mainly around the middle?	☐	☐
6. Do you have high blood pressure?	☐	☐
7. Is your cholesterol elevated?	☐	☐
8. Do you retain fluid?	☐	☐
9. Do you frequently crave sugar and/or starchy foods?	☐	☐
10. Do/Did either of your parents have adult-onset diabetes?	☐	☐

	Yes	No
11. Do/Did either of your parents have high blood pressure?	☐	☐
12. Does/Did one or more of your parents and/or grandparents have elevated triglycerides, elevated cholesterol, a heart attack, or gout?	☐	☐
13. Are you obese? (more than 20% overfat)	☐	☐

Scoring your health quiz:

Questions 1–5 If you answered "yes" to any of these questions, you already have, or are at very high risk of developing, an insulin-related disorder.

Questions 6–10 If you answered "yes" to any of these questions, you are at high risk of already having or developing an insulin-related disorder.

Questions 11–13 If you answered "yes" to any of these questions, you run a moderately high risk of having or developing an insulin-related disorder.

If you find that you're at risk, the low-carb diet is for you. Take a look at why it will work, or, if you're convinced and ready to go low-carb, dive in on page 24.

Food Was the Cause, Food Is the Solution

Just as food has gotten us into this dilemma, it will also get us out. Food—the right food—is the tool that will restore harmony to your harried metabolism. *The 30-Day Low-Carb Diet Solution* works because it feeds your body what it must have to thrive—protein from lean meat, fish, poultry, game, eggs, and dairy products; good fats found in olive oil, butter, coconut oil, nut oils, fish, and healthy, natural meat and poultry; antioxidants and cancer-fighting phytochemicals found in low-starch fruits, vegetables, and greens—and limits the grains, starchy fruits and vegetables, and sugars that are what's taking it out of balance. A low-carb diet is, in effect, a return to the kind of diet we were designed to thrive on over many millennia. The solution is so simple— give your body the nutritional tools it needs and then get out of its way and it will use these tools to heal you. In the first 30 days on this plan, you'll experience tremendous benefit both in weight loss and in reductions of blood pressure, blood sugar, cholesterol, and triglycerides.

What you eat will determine whether you store fat or burn it, make excess cholesterol and triglycerides or keep them in line, retain fluid or release it, elevate your blood pressure or keep it at a healthy level, suffer attacks of acid reflux or gout or don't. So it will pay great dividends to take just a moment to look briefly at what food is and how it affects you.

A Short Primer on Food

When you eat a meal, your body breaks down the food into its most basic units to make it possible to absorb the nutrients. No matter what you eat, all foods fall into three simple categories: protein, fat, and carbohydrate (starch, sugar, and fiber). And, of course, there's also water that makes up the lion's share of almost all foods.

The body breaks down protein, found mainly in meat, fish, poultry, eggs, dairy products, nuts, and tofu and other soy products, into individual amino acids that it reassembles and uses to build and repair body tissues—muscle, bone, blood, heart, liver, kidney, hair, skin, and nails—and to make all the enzymes and chemical messengers necessary to run virtually every process in the body.

Dietary fat, from both animal and vegetable sources, is assembled into absorbable clusters that pass first into the lymphatic system (a sort of superhighway of the immune system) and then into the blood. The body requires fat to make reproductive hormones (estrogen, testosterone, progesterone and others) and for proper function and maintenance of the brain, nervous system, and eyes, as well as a crucial component of the cell membrane of every one of the body's trillions of cells.

Most sugars, whether table sugar, fruit sugar, honey, syrups, or molasses, are all two simple sugar molecules—usually glucose and fructose—hooked together. Because the digestive tract quickly breaks these apart for absorption into the blood, they cause a quick rise in blood sugar, and for three-quarters of us that spells trouble. An exception is fructose (or the more-commonly used high-fructose corn syrup), which is absorbed differently. Fructose doesn't stimulate a rise in blood sugar and insulin and for years was thought of as a safe sugar for diabetics; however, research has clearly shown that it promotes insulin resistance by another mechanism and is therefore potentially the most dangerous and damaging of all the sugars.

Starches from corn, wheat, potatoes, rice, beans, and some fruits are nothing more than sugars in disguise. All starches are nothing more than lots of glucose (sugar) molecules hooked together in long chains. It is the business of your digestive system to break the links that hold the chains together so that you can absorb the simple sugar they contain. Starches are quickly broken into their most basic unit—glucose—and as a result they, too, can send your blood sugar through the roof. For example, eating a potato—just one good-sized potato—is the metabolic equivalent of eating a quarter of a cup of sugar. Once broken down to glucose, that potato will cause all the same reactions in your body as if you'd eaten a quarter of a cup of sugar. The same is true for other starchy foods, such as bread, crackers, muffins, waffles, pastries, pasta, rice, and to a lesser extent, dried beans and peas.

Fiber, like starch, is also made of long chains of sugar molecules hooked together, but the links are forged in a way that our digestive systems cannot break. Humans, unlike cows or other herbivores, have no means to extract the glucose from fiber; therefore, it cannot be absorbed into our blood or cause an increase in blood sugar or insulin.

Combined with other starches, fiber will help to slow down the absorption of sugars contained in any food, but not sufficiently to give you carte blanche to eat them. Although technically a carbohydrate (since it's made of sugars), fiber is a low-carb freebie, because we can't get to the sugar. From a practical standpoint, that means that when you're determining how much carbohydrate you can safely eat each day, you can ignore any amount contributed by fiber.

Food's Effect on Metabolism

Except for fiber and water, no food is free. There's a metabolic consequence to every bite you eat. It may be a good one, or it may be a disastrous one, but one thing is certain: when you eat, something's going to happen. If you hope to harness your metabolism and make it work for you instead of against you, it's important that you learn a few simple rules about what happens when you eat. How do the basic nutrient components of foods—protein, carbohydrate, and fat—influence the two crucial metabolic hormones, insulin and glucagon?

Carbohydrates cause metabolic havoc by sending insulin rapidly upward and causing glucagon to fall or remain unchanged. (It is actually the ratio between insulin and glucagon that determines the metabolic effect; the higher insulin goes and/or the lower glucagon falls, the more profound the effect.) Protein causes a modest, balanced rise in both insulin and glucagon, leading to no metabolic swing. Fat, fiber, and water have no effect on either insulin or glucagon—these foods are metabolically neutral. So the culprits in unhinging your metabolic control are clearly the sugars and starches in your diet. And it's by limiting these foods that you'll achieve the metabolic harmony that will restore your health and weight.

And therein lies the problem with the U.S. Department of Agriculture (USDA) food pyramid. Take a look at it in Figure 1. According

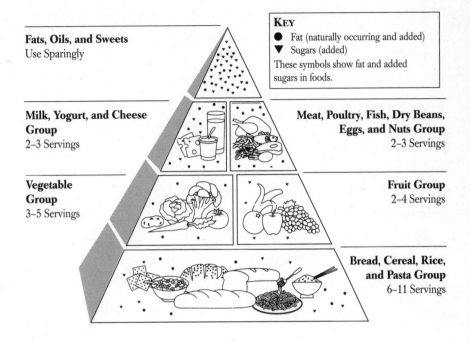

Fats, Oils, and Sweets
Use Sparingly

KEY
●   Fat (naturally occurring and added)
▼   Sugars (added)
These symbols show fat and added
sugars in foods.

**Milk, Yogurt, and Cheese
Group**
2–3 Servings

**Meat, Poultry, Fish, Dry Beans,
Eggs, and Nuts Group**
2–3 Servings

**Vegetable
Group**
3–5 Servings

Fruit Group
2–4 Servings

**Bread, Cereal, Rice,
and Pasta Group**
6–11 Servings

Figure 1. The USDA Food Pyramid

to the USDA recommendations, North Americans are supposed to be eating a diet of 60 percent carbohydrate, 15 percent protein, and 25 percent or less fat. Based on what you've just learned about the metabolic effect of foods, what effect would you expect to see? What effect does eating fat have on insulin? Zero, nada, zip! And what about protein from the meat, fish, poultry, eggs, and dairy the USDA recommends that you limit? It causes a balanced rise in insulin and glucagon (and thus no change in their ratio). But look at the big bottom of the pyramid—where it says six to eleven servings of bread, cereal, or pasta daily. What effect will eating all those carbohydrates have on your insulin level? They'll send it through the roof.

Despite the best intentions, the USDA reasoning was flawed: if too much insulin is the problem, how can recommending a diet that further increases insulin be the solution? Obviously, it can't. It's like pouring gasoline on a fire to put it out and wondering why the flames shoot higher. Have you been roasting on this bonfire? If so, you can step out now.

Food Pyramid or Feed Pyramid?

The fact that carbohydrates make you fatter may be recent news to you, but it's old hat to farmers. For centuries they have used carbohydrates to fatten their hogs and cattle. That got us to thinking: what exactly is the composition of the feed used to fatten livestock? We made a trip to our local farmer's cooperative to see, and here's what we found. Take a look at Figures 2 and 3. On the right is a pyramid construction of the protein, carbs, and fat in the feed farmers use to fatten hogs: 61% carbohydrate, 25% fat, and 14% protein. Compare it to the pyramid on the left—the USDA Food Pyramid—the one that you were told would keep you slim and healthy.

Look familiar? It should; the two are virtually identical. Now you see why the high-carbohydrate, low-fat diet fattened North America. So how much carbohydrate do our bodies really need? The answer may surprise you.

Although for years newspapers, magazines, and television talk shows have told you to load up on complex carbohydrates, like whole-

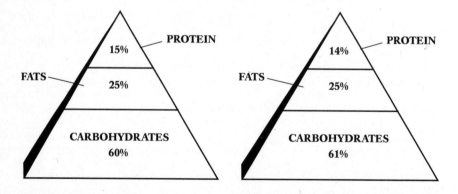

Figure 2. The USDA Food Pyramid   Figure 3. The Feed Lot Pyramid

grain breads, cereal, and pasta, because these foods form the basis of a healthy diet, your daily requirement for carbohydrate is actually *zero*. You read that right—none. Were you to make a search of all the textbooks in any medical library, although you will find diseases caused by both protein and essential fat deficiency, you will find no diseases of carbohydrate deficiency. That's why it has never made sense to us to load up on carbohydrates, which your body can use but doesn't really need, at the expense of fat and protein, which your body truly does need.

Why don't you need carbohydrate? Your body—actually your liver—has the ability to take dietary protein or fat (or your own body fat) and make glucose from it. The liver can make a couple of cups of sugar each day, which is more than enough to provide glucose for the few tissues in the body that prefer to use it. Most of the body, however, prefers to fuel itself with dietary or stored fat or with ketones (the natural break-down product of fat burning) instead of glucose.

Incredible as it may sound, you could do quite nicely without ever eating another bite of starch or sugar—as long as you had plenty of protein and fat. And that's just what all humans did for the three to four million years we were around prior to the advent of farming; we lived by hunting and fishing (the meat, poultry, and fish of our diets today) and gathering what grew wild: roots, shoots, nuts, and berries—and a bit of fruit in season. Not a bite of bread, cereal, rice, pasta, potatoes, or sugar.

Does that mean you should eat a diet without any carbohydrate? Not necessarily, but you could. And when you're initially working to correct your health, lose weight, control your blood sugar, or lower your cholesterol and triglycerides or blood pressure, you'll want to focus on limiting carbs more stringently. (You'll find all the details in chapter 2.) Critics of the low-carb approach have traditionally pointed to these lowest-carb corrective phases of the diet and decreed them to be too restrictive for long-term use. The irony is that you don't have to stay on them for the long term—they're merely an effective tool to correct the problem quickly. Once you near your goals (in weight or health) you can become more liberal with your carb limits, expand your intake of foods, and enjoy eating an even wider variety of fruits, vegetables, and even some higher-carb foods occasionally. Although an ultra-low-carb diet of fresh meat, fish, greens, and green veggies will provide all the essential vitamins and minerals needed for good health, it can become monotonous. Also, prolonged cooking of meat can rob it of the vitamin nutrients it contains. For these reasons, we encourage you to eat a wide variety of low-carb fruits, colorful vegetables, and greens for the beneficial vitamins, minerals, and cancer-fighting phytochemicals they contain. To take out all the guesswork, we've included 30 days' worth of meal plans to guide you, starting on page 44. As to the structure of what you'll be eating, if we were to create a Low-Carb Pyramid, it would look something like this:

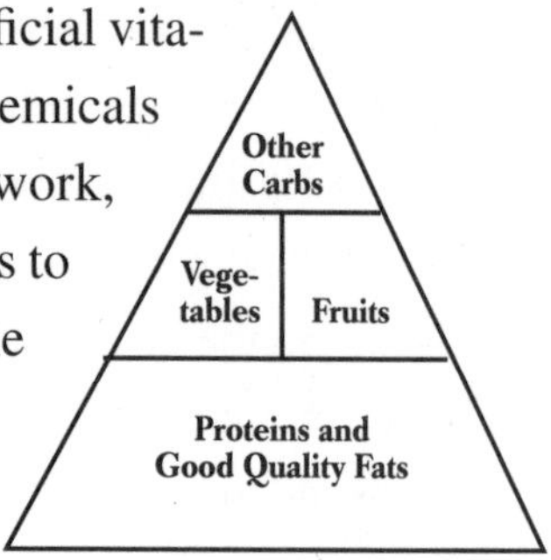

Figure 4. The Low-Carb Pyramid

The Health Benefits of Going Low-Carb
Lowering Cholesterol and Triglycerides

If you've been struggling with a low-fat diet, practically going no-fat in an effort to reduce your cholesterol, and not getting the results you want, you're in for a pleasant surprise. After using the low-carb approach for nearly twenty years to solve these problems for patients in our own clinic, we can guarantee that there's no safer or more effective way to lower your blood lipids. Take a look at this story from our case files:

Annie H.

Back in the mid-1980s, Annie came to our clinic complaining of abdominal discomfort. At thirty-four, and being a female, we suspected, based on her symptoms, that she might have gallstones and did some preliminary blood tests. Her lab work astonished us: a cholesterol reading of over 700 and triglycerides of nearly 3,000. Because she had not been fasting when we drew the blood and because the results were so incredibly high, we repeated the tests the next morning when she'd been without food overnight to be sure the report wasn't in error. On the second battery of tests, the cholesterol was about the same and triglycerides were even higher than before; an ultrasound test showed that, although she had a gall bladder full of sludge, she didn't have gallstones. Her abdominal discomfort came from the accumulation of fat in her liver, a common consequence of insulin resistance, even though she'd been following a low-fat diet for some time.

We began Annie on an ultra-low-carb diet of eggs, meat, fish, or chicken with green salad and green beans—along with plenty of water and a multivitamin with some supplemental potassium and magnesium. A restrictive low-carb prescription, to be sure, but also an effective one.[1] When we repeated her blood tests in three weeks (yes, you read that right, three weeks) her triglycerides had fallen to under 200 and her cholesterol had fallen into the normal range. And although she wasn't really overweight, she'd lost a few pounds to boot. At that point, we were able to begin to add a wider variety of foods to her very basic corrective diet, starting with more servings of green and colorful vegetables, such as peppers and summer squashes, along with nuts, cheese, melons, and berries. Then slightly-higher-carb fruits, such as oranges, peaches, plums, and starchier veggies, such as winter squash, carrots, and green peas. As she progressed into maintenance, she increased the portions of these nutrient-rich foods and was able to maintain her correction.

---

[1]If you are currently on medication to control blood sugar, blood pressure, or lipids, do not attempt an ultra-low-carb diet without first consulting your physician. Your need for these medications will be markedly reduced on such a plan and you will need to work with your physician to adjust your dosages as you diet. It is unwise and unsafe for you to adjust or discontinue medications on your own.

Why is a low-fat diet so ineffective for lowering cholesterol? Because, although it seems reasonable that cutting dietary fat and cholesterol should lower your cholesterol, in reality the fat you eat has very little to do with the fat level in your blood. Only about 20 percent of the cholesterol in your blood comes from the diet; the lion's share comes from within. Your own liver is a cholesterol production factory. The production line looks something like this: raw materials enter at one end, are altered in a series of steps, and the finished product—cholesterol—exits from the other end. The crucial step along the way—called the rate-limiting step—is under the control of (you guessed it) insulin.

When insulin levels are high, the liver is told to produce more cholesterol; bringing insulin levels down will decrease the production of cholesterol and significantly lower the amount in your blood. By following *The 30-Day Low-Carb Diet Solution,* you'll quickly bring your insulin levels down, and before long you'll be rewarded with a cholesterol reading in the normal range. The lowering of triglycerides comes about in a different way. Because their production is driven by eating sugar and starches or by excess alcohol consumption, reducing them simply means reducing the amount of sugar and starch you eat and cutting back the amount of alcohol you drink.

Long thought to be harmless, elevated triglycerides are now considered a major risk factor for the development of heart disease. Among our clinic patients we've found that the triglyceride levels along with the levels of the "good" HDL cholesterol are the most sensitive indicators of insulin resistance.

Raising Your "Good" HDL Cholesterol

For years, clinical research has shown that eating a low-fat diet will lower the level of "good" HDL cholesterol in your blood. Because HDL cholesterol exerts a protective effect against heart disease, low levels of HDL cholesterol—even in the absence of any other risk factors—are now considered a marker of heart disease risk.

Three things will raise your HDL: drinking moderately, exercising regularly, and eating good quality fats, such as those in nuts, seeds, olives, avocados, butter, and fish oil. All components, you'll notice, of a healthy low-carb diet—except the exercise, which is up to you to do.[2]

Reduced Risk of Heart Disease

Elevated insulin levels increase the risk of heart disease in a number of ways. You've just learned that excess insulin raises the level of cholesterol and triglycerides in the blood and decreases the levels of the good, protective HDL, all of which increase your risk of developing heart disease. But beyond its impact on lipids (the scientific term for cholesterol and fat in the blood), elevated insulin also causes the blood to be more prone to clot and the walls of the arteries that carry blood to the heart to thicken. Together, these two effects cause a decreased blood flow to the heart and a greater probability of blockage formation. And in addition, elevated insulin stimulates a cascade of inflammation that new research is showing may be the root cause of heart disease. Take a look at Mitch J.'s story.

Mitch J.

Mitch was driving along the interstate one day in 1996, half listening to an NPR radio interview we were giving from a small radio station in his area. The interviewer asked us how we could square the fact that while we said our fat-and-protein–rich, low-carb diet reduced the risk

---

[2]For detailed information about what we feel is the best kind of exercise to keep you lean and healthy in a program that will only take thirty minutes a week, pick up a copy of our book, *The Slow-Burn Fitness Revolution.*

of heart disease, Dr. Dean Ornish claimed that his very-low-fat, near-vegetarian diet (virtually the opposite diet to ours) could do the same? Mitch was mildly interested in hearing our answer to this, since he had keeled over with a heart attack while running a year or so before while traveling abroad. (He'd been a regular, avid runner for many years.) Subsequent to his heart attack, his cardiologist had put him on the Ornish diet to restore his health, and he truly believed he was doing the prudent thing by following what is for most people an extremely boring and tasteless diet. He was almost laughing to himself, wondering how we could possibly answer that question.

We answered with facts. In the data from Dr. Ornish's own published reports on patients following his plan, in each and every instance, their triglycerides went up and their HDL went down. Based on these two major indicators of heart disease risk, all his patients actually *increased* their risk for having another heart attack. That got Mitch's attention; he cranked up the volume and pulled off onto the shoulder of the road to listen intently. He'd just gotten his most recent lab report showing exactly that result: HDL falling and triglycerides up to such a level that his doctor was talking about putting him on medication to bring it down.

Still skeptical, Mitch bought a copy of our book, *Protein Power,* and being of a scientific bent, he plowed through the medical research and the scientific underpinnings and decided to give it a try. In short order, he lost a little weight, his triglycerides plummeted, and his HDL rose into the healthy range. Almost seven years later, now retired from his medical practice, he's still faithfully following his plan and is able to ski circles around his much younger friends each winter. Can this diet reverse heart disease? You bet.

Preserving Your Lean Body

Have you ever known someone who lost a fair amount of weight on a low-fat low-calorie diet? More than likely, they looked haggard and gaunt, with sagging, pasty skin and lackluster hair. This haggard appearance comes from not eating enough good quality protein to rebuild the tissues that break down normally, just from living.

Because it also requires protein to manufacture important chemicals, enzymes, and messengers, when there's not enough protein coming in through the diet to do the job, the body will begin to consume itself, breaking down its muscles and lean organs for the raw materials it needs. Self-preservation dictates that it will begin with the least important muscles. So the facial muscles go early on, giving the face a sagging older appearance. Not far behind are the shoulder and arm muscles. By the time the diet is over, the supportive infrastructure is lost and the skin just seems to hang on the frame.

Maybe you've seen that happen or even fear your weight loss will make you look and feel older than you are. Don't worry. If you carefully follow the easy nutritional plan outlined for you in *The 30-Day Low-Carb Diet Solution* you'll always have plenty of good quality protein to preserve even the small muscles of your face. Like many of our patients, your friends will soon be asking what new facial care system or cosmetic wonder you've found that's making you look ten years younger.

Cheryl's Story

Cheryl's parents brought her to us, deeply concerned about her weight. At only 17 years old and just 5'4" tall, Cheryl already weighed almost 250 pounds. Beyond their concerns for her health, her mom and dad felt that the excess weight had begun to interfere with her participation in the fun activities a girl her age should enjoy. We evaluated her and felt that their concerns were indeed well-founded and that she could benefit tremendously from a low-carb diet. We had our doubts, however, about whether going on our diet program was Cheryl's idea or her parents. In the latter case, nutritional intervention almost never succeeds, no matter how effective the program. Quite simply, the person doing the dieting must be the person who wants to attain the goal. As much as parents may want their overweight children to lose, unless the children want it for themselves, it will simply not work. After many years of experience, we can attest that the best way to get overweight children or teens to lose weight is to provide a good example yourself, make good nutrition available at home, do family activities that encourage fitness, and don't harp on the issue of weight.

Cheryl assured us that she was ready to go, and we started her on the diet. By two weeks, she was off the wagon. She complained that the food made her sick to her stomach; she didn't like the taste of this or that; she just couldn't stay with it. And that was that.

About two years later—at age 19—Cheryl returned to us on her own. By this time, she'd ballooned to 309 pounds, had already developed high blood pressure, was puffing and panting just to walk, and had to be helped up onto the exam table. After a second evaluation more ominous than the first, we started Cheryl on the diet again. And this time, she loved the food, enjoyed her protein shakes in the morning, and had no trouble sticking with the plan. After a little over a year, she was down to 135 pounds! The day she came into the clinic in her younger sister's miniskirt, she was beaming and bursting to tell us about her new boyfriend—her first one ever.

You'll hear from critics of the low-carb diet that all the weight you lose is water. If that were the case, Cheryl must have been just a big water balloon! The truth is that when you eat properly on a low-carb plan, you do lose a little water at first, but mainly you lose body fat. At the same time, the rich protein intake helps to preserve your lean muscles. Despite having ballooned to over 300 pounds and then having lost over 170 pounds, Cheryl looked fantastic in that black miniskirt— lean, strong, trim, and most important, healthy. If Cheryl can do it, so can you.

Controlling Blood Sugar

Diabetes afflicts an estimated 16 million North Americans, with another 16 million or so hovering on the border, about to become diabetic. Once a disease of adulthood, type II diabetes (the kind associated with insulin resistance and excess insulin in the blood) now turns up in second graders. For years diabetic nutritional counselors have put their patients on the standard American Diabetic Association low-fat diet, containing 60 percent carbohydrate or more. Diabetes is a disease of too much sugar in the blood, so how can putting even more sugar in the blood help? The answer, of course, is that it doesn't, whether you put it in as broken-down starch or as sugar itself, it's all going to raise the blood sugar.

There is no more effective way to lower elevated blood sugar than to quit adding fuel to the fire—simply cut back on rich sources of carbohydrate and blood sugar will usually fall into the normal range in short order.

A word of caution: If you are diabetic and currently taking medication to lower your blood sugar, do not begin the corrective phase of this program without discussing it with your physician. This program lowers blood sugar so effectively that, in combination with your medication, your blood sugar could become dangerously low. You must work with your physician to reduce and/or discontinue diabetic medications as you progress. It is not safe for you to attempt to reduce or discontinue your own medications.

Remember the Nutritional Pop Quiz at the start of the chapter? Every statement there is true; how did you score?

Now that you're better versed in how going low-carb will help you, let's get you started on *The 30-Day Low-Carb Diet Solution.*

CHAPTER 2

Getting Ready to Go Low-Carb

You're going to be amazed at how quickly and effortlessly a low-carb diet restores your health and fitness. In a matter of days you'll feel the difference—more energy, less hunger—and in a matter of a few weeks you'll experience dramatic reductions in blood pressure, blood sugar, or lipids if they're elevated. We encourage you to get a pre-diet snapshot of your current health: see your physician for a physical exam, ask for a check of your blood pressure, blood sugar, blood lipids, height, and weight.

As a pleasant side benefit, you'll lose excess body fat. In order to optimize the potency of a low-carb diet, simply remember these two cardinal rules:

1. **Always meet your daily protein requirement**
2. **Never exceed your carbohydrate limit per meal or per day**

In order to follow even that simple plan, however, you'll need to determine the amounts of protein and carbohydrate that are right for you—and doing that has never been easier. All you'll need to know are three things: your height, your weight[1], and your gender.

Finding Your Protein Requirement

Armed with those three simple pieces of information, turn to the appropriate table in Appendix D (women on page 176 and men on page 177). Find your height across the top of the table and your weight (rounded to the nearest five pounds) down the left-hand side. Draw a line down from your height and another line across from your weight; where the two intersect, you'll find your general protein requirement—it will be small (S), medium (M), large (L), extra-large (X) or extra-extra-large (XX). You'll find the selection of foods you will eat to meet each of these daily protein intakes in the Protein Servings Lists on pages 58 to 60. This will give you a good idea of what you should aim for in portion sizes. Simply select any item from the list that fits your size requirement and that will be an appropriate serving of protein for you—pick one of these for each of your three meals a day and you'll be sure to get enough protein. You can even throw in an additional protein snack for good measure if you like.

For most people (certainly for most men) it's sufficient simply to say: eat all the protein foods you want. Eat of them until you're full and satisfied. Make sure you get enough, but don't worry about going over your allotment of protein. Don't worry about weighing and measuring, just eat what you want of steak, prime rib, chicken, fish, lobster, hamburger, nuts, cheese, eggs, and bacon—any of the foods on the protein list—and enjoy. The health corrections seen with low-carb eating will occur virtually independent of calorie intake, as long as you keep carbs controlled. (And incredibly, most people with weight to lose will lose it easily—seemingly no matter how much of these foods they eat.) However, if you're trying to lose weight and are not losing or you were losing but hit a plateau, simply become a bit more mind-

---

[1]In order to optimize your results, you should really weigh and measure yourself to be certain of your correct height and weight.

ful of sticking closer to your protein target and your weight loss should resume.

Sometimes Calories Do Count

For smaller people—especially for women, but for men of small stature as well—portion size matters more when weight loss is a goal. To optimize your weight loss on *The 30-Day Low-Carb Diet Solution*, it's best both to spread your food intake out throughout the day and to stick reasonably close to your target protein intake and even to select protein sources that are a bit leaner. Most good sources of complete protein are also good sources of fat and, therefore, of calories.

When you're small, it simply doesn't take as many calories to run your body each day as it would someone larger. Although limiting carbs sets the metabolic stage to make it easier for you to lose fat, unless your body needs the calories you've stored in your fat cells, it won't go to the trouble of bringing them out and burning them. Only when you're eating fewer calories than it takes to meet your daily energy needs will your body turn to its fat stores. And for this reason, small people have to be somewhat mindful of calories as well as carbs when they're trying to lose weight.

It will also be more important for a smaller person to try to eat more often. Eating three smaller meals a day, instead of one huge one, smoothes the metabolic response to the food, keeps insulin levels in tighter check, and makes weight loss easier. Don't stress too much about it, though; it's okay to have a little less protein at one meal (breakfast, for instance) and a little more at another, or only get your requirement in two somewhat larger servings on some days. Your body is metabolically well equipped to juggle these meal-to-meal or day-to-day protein differences. That said, no matter how big or small you are, you will still see the best results from spreading out your intake.

Why Is Protein So Important?

The human body is mainly made of protein; your hair, skin, nails, blood, bones, muscles, organs, ligaments, immune system, nerves—all of them—are made of protein. Just in the course of living, these tissues break down, wear out, and must be regularly replaced and repaired. To do that job, you must provide your body with a steady supply of high-quality protein.

In our practice, we often saw patients skimp on their protein servings in the mistaken belief that fewer calories (of any kind) would make them lose weight faster. Clearly calories do matter, but when you're trying to encourage your body to burn stored fat, skimping on protein foods works against you for three important reasons:

Protein keeps your metabolic rate high. Because the body understands that protein is its most critical nutrient, it keys its metabolic rate (the number of calories it uses each day) to the amount of protein it receives.

Protein satisfies your appetite, as well. Research has shown that the meal interval—the length of time your appetite is satisfied between meals—depends on the quality and the quantity of the protein of your most recent meal.

Protein preserves your lean body mass—the part of you that uses calories. The more your lean body weighs, the more calories it takes in a day to run it. If you skimp on protein, you may lose some of these metabolically active, calorie-using pounds. That's weight loss, certainly, but not the kind you want; for good health and easier maintenance of your goal weight, you want to lose only excess fat.

Cutting the Carbs

Since carbohydrates control your insulin and insulin controls your metabolic health, here's where the rubber meets the road in low-carb dieting.

To correct a metabolism run amok (and the excess weight, blood sugar, blood pressure, cholesterol, triglycerides, or other health problems that come about because of it) you'll want to carefully control your carbohydrate intake at each meal throughout the day—particularly in the beginning. As your weight drops and your health improves, you'll be able to graduate to eating bigger servings of a wider variety of foods and still maintain your health and fitness. So how much carb can you eat? To find out, answer a few simple questions:

	Yes	No
1. Do you need to lose more than 20 percent of your total body weight?	☐	☐
2. Do you have high blood pressure?	☐	☐
3. Do you have diabetes?	☐	☐
4. Do you have elevated cholesterol or triglycerides?	☐	☐
5. Do you have sleep apnea?	☐	☐
6. Do you have acid reflux?	☐	☐
7. Are you on medications for any of these conditions?[2]	☐	☐

If you answered no to *all* of questions 1 through 6, you will begin with Moderate Carbohydrate Servings (page 63) at each meal and snack and remain there until you approach your target weight or health goals, then move to Large Carbohydrate Servings (page 66) for the long term.

If you answered yes to *any* of questions 1 through 6, you will begin with Small Carbohydrate Servings (page 60) at each meal or snack and remain at this level until you approach your target weight and have resolved your health concerns. It may seem difficult at first to limit

---

[2]If you are currently under a physician's care or take prescription medication for any condition, please check with your physician before beginning this or any diet.

your carb intake to small servings, but it helps to think of the many benefits that you'll gain: not only will you be losing body fat and looking better, but you'll be doing wonders for your blood pressure, cholesterol, blood sugar, and heart. This one simple change—cutting back on your intake of carbohydrates—will do more for your health and well being than just about anything else could.

> If you answered yes to question 7, although the Small Carbohydrate Limit will be the correct one for you initially, you should not begin the diet until you're able to work with your physician to reduce the dosages of your medications. This diet is a powerful tool that will reduce blood pressure and blood sugar quickly—if you are taking medications to reduce them as well, your blood sugar or pressure could drop dangerously low. Your physician will be able to reduce (and in most cases discontinue) these medications as your new diet heals you, but you must not attempt to do this on your own. It's less critical to immediately adjust medications that control blood lipids or acid reflux, although these, too, will likely become a thing of the past soon.

What About Fats?

There's no need to stringently restrict fats on a low-carb diet the same way you must carbohydrates. Instead, incorporate them sensibly and stick as much as possible to good natural fats and oils, such as:

Olive oil

Nut oils: walnut, macadamia, hazelnut, almond

Peanut oil

Sesame seed oil

Avocado oil

Butter

Coconut oil

Oils from cold-water fish (salmon, sardines, mackerel, herring, tuna) and cod liver oil

Lard from naturally raised animals

Of course, some of the fat in your diet will also come from the delicious foods these oils are derived from: olives, avocados, nuts, seeds, seafood, meat, and dairy products.

For best health, you'll want to stay away from the partially hydrogenated oils: corn oil, vegetable oils (including safflower, sunflower, soybean, and canola oils), vegetable shortening, and margarine. All these products contain *trans* fats—altered fat molecules that have been reported to be the unhealthiest fats, suspected to promote obesity, heart disease, cancer, diabetes, and a host of other ills.

What to Expect in 30 Days

On this 30-day low-carb plan your health parameters, such as blood sugar, blood pressure, and lipids, should correct completely—or nearly so—almost no matter how out of line they currently are. If you've got a lot of weight to lose, however, you probably won't have reached your weight goals in 30 days, but you'll be well on your way. If you're a man, our experience tells us you will lose an average of 3 to 5 pounds of fat a week following a corrective low-carb diet—it's often a bit faster in the first few weeks, but it will level out to about this average over the long haul. If you're a woman, you can expect to lose an average of 2 to 4 pounds per week—usually also a little faster at first. That means that in 30 days, on average, men following a corrective low-carb diet can realistically expect to lose 12 to 20 pounds of fat and women about 8 to 16 pounds. To lose weight, you've got to burn up the excess storage, and, no matter how you slice it, this takes time. The more storage there is, the more time it takes. At 15 to 20 pounds a month, simple math tells you it will take a couple of months to drop 30 or 40 pounds, five to six months to drop 100. But you won't get thinner any sooner any other way.

The 30-Day Low-Carb Diet Solution eliminates all the guesswork about what to eat. You'll find 30 days of complete meal plans, beginning on page 44, to guide you each day through breakfast, lunch, dinner, and an optional snack. With these in hand, you're set to begin. They're arranged to begin at the lower end of the carb scale and to progress by the end of the 30 days to a slightly more moderate level.[3] We've even added a very basic, generic plan that you can use to guide you when you dine out, or as a template to build your own low-carb meal plans.

If you elect not to use the meal plans provided in this book, don't forget the two cardinal rules:

Always meet your daily protein requirement
Never exceed your carbohydrate limit per meal or per day

Remember that, although your protein intake is a minimum requirement and in most cases you can have a bigger serving if you would like it, the same is not true for carbs. Because of the metabolic consequence of eating starches and sugars, your carbohydrate portion is a maximum you should try not to exceed—especially during the corrective phase of your low-carb diet. Remember, too, that you won't be in the corrective phase forever—just until you correct your problems. With time, you'll be able to substantially increase the amounts and variety of the carb-containing foods you eat.

---

[3]If you're beginning at the Moderate level, you can simply make the fruit and veggie servings of the meal plans a little bigger if you like. For guidance on how big, refer to the Moderate Carbohydrate Servings List on page 63.

How Will You Know When to Graduate to More Carbs?

We recommend that for best results during the corrective phase of your diet you keep your total daily carbohydrate intake at the Small level (about 10 grams of effective carbohydrate[4] per meal or a total of 30 to 40 grams of effective carbohydrate each day).

Once you near your target weight and have corrected any associated health problems, you'll graduate to a richer carb intake, both per meal and per day. During this transition period, increase your carbohydrate intake to the Moderate level (about 15 grams of effective carbohydrate per meal or snack, for a total of 50 to 60 grams of effective carbohydrate each day).

If you're able to maintain your correction on the Moderate level of carbohydrates for several weeks, graduate to the Large level (about 20 grams of effective carbohydrate in each meal or snack, for a total of 60 to 80 grams of effective carbohydrate each day).

Finally, if your correction holds at the Large level of carbohydrate grams for a few weeks, you can safely remain on this level for the long term. At that point, you can mix and match carb servings from all the lists to inch your daily intake even higher—as long as eating more carbs doesn't adversely affect your health, weight, or fitness. Everyone will have a carb limit—some higher than others. Your limit is the amount you can eat each day and not regain your weight; see your blood pressure, blood sugar, or lipid readings begin to climb again; or see your GE reflux, gout, or sleep apnea return. Now let's look at what you'll be eating on your new low-carb diet.

---

[4]Effective carbohydrate content (ECC) is the term we developed to describe the actual amount of usable sugars and starches in a given food. It is the grams of total carbohydrate content minus the grams of fiber, sugar alcohols, or other nonabsorbable or partially absorbable carbohydrates in a food. All carb listings here are given as EC grams. Pick up a copy of *The Protein Power LifePlan Gram Counter* for a handy reference—available at bookstores nationwide or online.

CHAPTER 3

So . . . What Do I Eat?

Figuring out what to eat on a low-carb diet can be as simple as our son, Ted, used to make it: *Just don't eat white things.* That simple admonition leaves all the meats, fish, poultry, and colorful fruits and veggies on your plate, but cuts out flour, sugar, potatoes, breads, pastries, pasta, rice, dried beans, bananas—the white things that one and all are high in starch or sugar. Unfortunately, the nothing-white dictum would also eliminate cauliflower, egg whites, cream, many cheeses, and yogurt—all "good" white things that a low-carb diet would allow. Moreover, that scheme would leave in such things as corn, which is yellow, but quite high in starch (since it's actually a grain and not a vegetable), as well as a raspberry Slurpee, which isn't white either (although the sugar that sweetens it is), but which isn't going to do your insulin level any favors. However, if you apply it with common sense, this simple rule will serve as a pretty good guide of what to eat when you go low-carb.

You could also adopt the slightly different version of this guideline coined by one of our readers: *If it's white, better go light. If it's colorful or brown, wolf it down.* That works pretty well, too—with the same admonitions about the cauliflower, egg whites, dairy products, and corn—but, again, only if you're applying it to whole foods and not to confections. Among the latter, you'd find chocolate cake, pinto beans, and pumpernickel rye in the brown category and the aforementioned raspberry Slurpee in with the sweet potatoes in the colorful one. Not to mention strawberry mousse and peach ice cream, which unless you're making our *Low-Carb Comfort Food Cookbook*[1] versions of these breads and treats, would be full of those proscribed white things, sugar and flour, and would send your blood sugar and insulin through the roof. So, again, apply this simple scheme with a serving of common sense—even if it's red or purple or plaid, if a big dose of white (sugar or flour) hides within it, consider it white!

Another patient once offered a more straightforward, but stringently purist guide to what to eat on a low-carb diet: *If you could hunt it with a spear or gather it in the woods 20,000 years ago, you can eat it!* And, indeed, if you ever have a question about what to eat to be absolutely, positively sure you're eating a healthy low-carb meal, that scheme will never fail you. You can't go wrong eating anything that falls into either of those categories. But there are too many deliciously wonderful foods available to us nowadays to be so restrictive, and you really don't have to be that much of a purist to enjoy the many health benefits of going low-carb.

If you're following a low-carb diet just to stay healthy—i.e., you don't need to lose weight and you have no health issues, such as elevated cholesterol, triglycerides, blood pressure, or blood sugar that you need to correct—just eat as much as you want of the foods listed here and don't concern yourself with amounts. If you do have corrections to make, follow the simple guidelines we've outlined in Chapter 2, Getting Ready to Go Low-Carb.

Now, let's look at what's cookin' in a low-carb kitchen.

---

[1]*The Low-Carb Comfort Food Cookbook* (Wiley, 2003) contains over three hundred recipes for delicious low-carb breads, pies, cakes, muffins, pasta, pizza—even fried chicken—to make going low-carb easier than ever.

What to Eat: Getting Your Protein

You can meet your protein requirement with meats, fish, poultry, game, eggs, nuts, dairy products or whey-, egg-, or soy-based[2] protein powders. All of these are sources of complete protein. If you choose, you can also use soybeans, tofu, TVP, and soymilk. (You'll find the complete Protein Servings Lists on pages 58–60 for small, medium, large, extra-large, and double-extra-large portions to give you an idea of how much protein you should be aiming for in a meal.)

It's important to remember that while meat, fish, poultry, game, and eggs are mainly protein and fat and have little or no carbohydrate, dairy protein sources (cheeses, cream, milk, yogurt, whey), nuts, and vegetable protein sources (soy products and nuts) all contain some undercover carbs, as well as the protein and fat. Not much in the case of cheeses, cream, whey, and nuts, but enough in fluid milk, yogurt, and some soy products that you at least need to be mindful of them during the corrective phase of your diet. We've included a helpful list, the Carbohydrate Content of Combination Foods (page 169) to help guide your choices.

What to Eat: What is a Carb, Anyway?

When people first begin a low-carb diet, there's often a bit of confusion about exactly what a carbohydrate is. The short answer is that it is the sugar, starch, or fiber in a food—and remember, starch is nothing more than the storage form of sugar. In general, you'll find carbohydrates in any food that is a fruit, a vegetable, or a grain.

Many foods or food products are made primarily of carbohydrate: sugar, flour, cereal grains, such as rice, corn, wheat, oats, and all the

---

[2]Medical research has begun to show that processed soy—such as is found in soy protein powders, some tofu, soy flours, soymilk, and texturized vegetable proteins used to make *faux* meat products—may be harmful to health. Although the jury is still out, our best current advice is to use these sparingly if at all.

foods made from these things—bread, cereal, muffins, cookies, cakes, pies, crackers, chips, pasta, rice cakes—you get the picture. Apart from the starch or sugar they contain, these foods don't really offer much in the way of important nutrition unless they're fortified. But you'll find carbohydrate-rich foods in the fruit and veggie world as well, particularly in bananas, mango, papaya, potatoes, and yams. You'll find a list of carbohydrate servings for the small, moderate, and large serving sizes in Carbohydrate Serving Sizes on pages 60–70, but first, let's look at the kinds of carbohydrate-containing foods you'll be eating on a low-carb diet.

The Fruit Bowl

The carb content of fruits comes from the fruit sugar and fiber they contain—and there's quite a range. Among the many kinds of fruit you can enjoy on a low-carb diet, you'll find the best carb bargains in melons, cherries and berries, followed by grapes, and small peaches, plums, and oranges. Virtually any fruit is fair game, but to be permissible on a low-carb plan, the serving size for some of the higher carb ones may be pretty small, at least during the corrective (earliest) stage of the diet.

Eat: melons, berries, cherries, grapes, small peaches, plums, tangerines, and oranges.

Watch out for: fruit juices, bananas and other tropical fruits. And keep servings of apples or pears small at first.

The Vegetable Bin

The vegetable world, for the most part, is a kinder, gentler place to begin a low-carb plan. Here, you'll find a wealth of foods rich in nutrition, low in starch, and high in fiber. Of course, there are a few vegetables that are high in carbs as well, and you'll want to limit or avoid those, particularly at first.

Eat: artichokes, asparagus, beets, black soybeans, broccoli, cabbage, cauliflower, cucumbers, green beans, collard, turnip, or mustard greens, lettuces, mushrooms, okra, peppers, spinach, sprouts, squashes, tomatoes, and turnips.

Beware of: corn, dried peas and beans, lentils, potatoes, and yams—these vegetables are high in starch and low in fiber and carry a significant carbohydrate load in the serving sizes you're probably accustomed to eating.

Because starch is just a chain of sugars that your body quickly breaks apart, you can think of the starch content of any food as its sugar equivalent. A large-sized baked potato, for instance, contains almost 50 grams of usable potato starch—an amount that when broken down by your digestive system equals about ¼ cup of sugar! You'd never dream of piling a quarter of a cup of sugar on your dinner plate alongside your steak, but that's in essence what you'd be doing with the potato. On the other hand, a one-cup serving of broccoli only has about 4 grams of usable carbohydrate—equivalent to less than a teaspoon of sugar. That's a much better option, if controlling insulin to lose excess weight and reclaim your health on a low-carb plan is your goal. If you really, really want the potato taste, do as we do: scrape out as much of the flesh as you can, toss it away, and then load up the skin with the butter, sour cream, chives, and bacon bits and enjoy for under 10 grams of carb.

What About the Fat?

In regard to fat, you should concern yourself with quality more than with quantity. The fat that you eat basically becomes *you*—it's incorporated into your brain, your nerve coverings, your eyes, and the delicate membrane of every single cell in your body. Because fat is essential for life and for good health, it behooves you to be serious about the kinds of fat that you eat.

Remember, however, that even though fats and oils don't raise your blood sugar or insulin—and contrary to the prevailing wisdom will *not* raise your cholesterol or triglycerides unless you eat a lot of carb with them[3]—they are a significant source of calories. If weight loss is a goal for you and if you're not losing or have stalled in your progress, keep a watchful eye on the quantity of fat as well as the quality until you've reached your target weight.

You'll want to choose from these good quality sources of fat, both for cooking and eating on this plan:

For salad dressings:

- Avocado oil
- Nut oils—walnut, macadamia, hazelnut, and almond
- Olive oil—extra-virgin or virgin, or pure if it's unadulterated by other oils
- Sesame oil

For Baking or Frying:

- Butter
- Coconut oil
- Olive oil*
- Peanut oil
- Sesame oil*
- Lard

*Use these oils for sautéing or frying at low temperatures only.

Drink Up

When you follow a low-carb plan, you don't retain excess fluid, making it even more important to keep yourself well hydrated. So how much should you drink? The simple answer is to drink as much water

[3]For all the science that backs up this assertion, pick up a copy of *The Protein Power LifePlan*.

or calorie-free (and aspartame free, preferably) fluid that you can. We recommend that you drink at least two quarts (sixty-four ounces) of noncalorie fluid a day.

Drinking water will help you remove excess ketones (the normal by-products of fat burning) from your system. While ketones are not harmful (in fact they're the preferred energy-producing fuel for the heart muscle), if you're breaking down more than you can use, they can cause a bit of insomnia, sometimes headache, and "ketone breath," a sharp fruity odor best overcome by drinking more water.

Although water is your best fluid option, don't feel you're limited to water alone. Any fluid that doesn't have calories is fair game. That includes diet soda[4], coffee (with or without caffeine), tea, and still or sparkling water.

Sweetening the Pot

Beware the use of excessive amounts of artificial sweeteners—for example, drinking one diet soda after the next—since the intense sweet taste can trick your body into believing that sugar has come in and stimulate the release of insulin, which can drop your blood sugar and make you hungry again. In the long run, artificial sweeteners may cause you to overeat. For some people, the same can be true for caffeine. If you find that you still have between-meal hunger pangs or that you're still retaining some fluid, you may want to consider cutting back on artificial sweeteners and caffeine.

When you do choose to use an artificial sweetener, do so in moderation. We recommend the use of sucralose (Splenda), acesulfame (Sweet One), saccharine (Sweet 'n' Low and others), or stevia leaf (Stevia Plus), but not aspartame (Equal and others).

---

[4]We can no longer recommend the use of products containing aspartame on a low-carb diet. Recent studies have shown that it may be harmful to the brain. For the complete details, see *The Protein Power LifePlan.*

Nutritional Insurance

A varied low-carb diet that includes meat, fish, seafood, poultry, eggs, and dairy, as well as plenty of berries, other fruits, and green and colorful vegetables will provide you with the recommended daily intakes of all the important vitamins, minerals, antioxidants, and phytochemicals necessary to keep you healthy. If you eat a wide selection of these foods regularly, fine. However, people do have food likes and dislikes, the availability of some fresh foods may vary seasonally or geographically, and the nutrient quality of canned or frozen items varies tremendously. Consequently, we have always recommended that our patients and readers avail themselves of an extra measure of nutritional insurance: a daily complete multivitamin and chelated mineral supplement (without iron[5]) and an additional supplement of magnesium and potassium.[6] You may be able to find a good quality product in a health and nutrition store near you, however, recent studies of a wide selection of these health food store products revealed that some of them contained little or none of what the label claimed. We've included the profile of what to look for in a good supplement product in Appendix B, page 173, as well as a resource for obtaining them by mail in the event that you're unable to find a similar product in your area.

Fruit of the Vine: Wine, Beer, and Spirits

Alcohol (beer, wine, or distilled spirits) is certainly permissible on a low-carb plan, as long as you use it sensibly. In these beverages, much

---

[5]Unless your physician has diagnosed you with iron deficiency, you should avoid taking extra iron in supplements. For the full details of the dangers of iron overload, see *The Protein Power LifePlan.*

[6]The over-the-counter varieties of these supplements usually provide a bit less than 100 mg of each per tablet. You should aim for taking about 400 mg of each of these minerals—or four over-the-counter tablets—per day.

of the sugar content has been fermented into alcohol and so the carb content is pretty low. Dry wines, for instance, contain about a gram of carb in each ounce—so 3 to 4 grams in the typical serving of wine. In moderation—a glass of a pert little pinot grigio or a full-bodied big cab or red zin at dinner—wine can not only improve your weight loss, but is also good for your heart as well. So enjoy, if you desire.

The carb cost is roughly the same for beer—about a gram or two per ounce, depending on its heaviness, with pale ales and pilsners on the low end and lagers and stouts on the high end. Unfortunately, however, a standard beer serving is 12 ounces and that adds up to 12 to 24 grams of carb or more. In the earliest stages of a low-carb correction, that's a pretty heavy hit on the carb scale. The good news is that if you're a beer drinker, lite beers can be your salvation; you can have a Miller Lite, Coors Light, or Pearl Light for about 3 or 4 grams of carb or an Amstel Light or Sam Adams Light for about 5 or 6 grams, so all is not lost.

In distilled spirits (bourbon, scotch, vodka, gin, tequila, brandy) the carbohydrate has mostly been turned to alcohol, so the actual carb count for an ounce of these liquors is negligible. What's not, however, is their elevating effect on your insulin and triglyceride levels, and potentially your weight—there are a lot of calories in them. Use discretion—a little is good, too much is often counterproductive.

Three Squares and Then Some

You don't have to limit yourself to three meals a day, although that's fine to do if you're comfortable with that. However, it's also okay to have a snack between breakfast and lunch or lunch and dinner or whenever you feel the need. In fact, in the beginning, we recommend that you plan on eating a little snack at least once a day. Not a candy, chips, or donut snack (unless you make these treats from *The*

Low-Carb Comfort Food Cookbook), but something nutritious: a handful of nuts, some cheese, deli meat, jerky, or leftover steak or chicken, with a cluster of grapes, a few juicy strawberries, or a small peach, plum, or tangerine, for instance. Even a low-carb protein bar or a protein shake can make a good, quick meal or snack on the run.

An important component to success with a low-carb diet is never to let yourself get hungry, when you'll be tempted to eat whatever comes to hand—even if it's a Twinkie. Keeping your blood sugar and insulin levels stable is a goal best served by eating smaller meals more frequently and sticking to real food or any of the dozens of delicious low-carb treats you can make yourself from our cookbook.

Making Substitutions

Because everyone has food preferences—likes, dislikes, allergies—you may find that you need or want to substitute certain foods for others on the meal plans. There's no reason that you can't do so within groups on the Protein Servings and Carbohydrate Servings lists. Within the carbohydrate group, you can substitute fruits for vegetables or bread/cereal/grain and vice versa as long as you stay at the same size carbohydrate serving—i.e., small for small, moderate for moderate, and large for large.

Here are some basic substitutions you may find helpful:

Berries can be interchanged easily. For instance, strawberries, blackberries, and raspberries are roughly equal in carbohydrate amounts and blueberries and boysenberries are about equal in carb content.

All the melons (cantaloupe, watermelon, and honeydew) have a similar carb content per cup.

Broccoli, cauliflower, asparagus and green beans are all about the same per cup.

Oranges, peaches, plums and tangerines all carry about the same carb load for a medium piece of fruit. Pears and apples are close in carb value and are interchangeable.

Within the squash families you can substitute the summer varieties—yellow (crookneck), zucchini, scallop, and spaghetti squash—across the board. The same is true for the winter varieties—acorn, butternut, and Hubbard.

If You Fall Off the Wagon: How to Recover

Chances are, before beginning a low-carb diet, you had been eating metabolically unsound foods for many years. Because these old eating habits die hard, we expect that on occasion you will fall off the wagon—after all, you're only human. Whether it's simply a one-time indulgence of an irresistibly sweet dessert while dining out or a full week's carb blow-out while you're on vacation, the trick is to get right back on the wagon as soon as possible.

Besides leaving you feeling somewhat guilty about your dietary diversion, don't be surprised if your fall off the wagon leaves you feeling sluggish, weak, and maybe even a few pounds heavier (mostly from fluid retention). The sooner you get back on track, the sooner you'll start feeling fit and healthy again—immediately return to the corrective level of this plan and remain there until you are back to the weight you were before the fall.

These excursions from the straight and narrow should be few and far between if you pick up a copy of our recently published book, *The Low-Carb Comfort Food Cookbook*. In it, we'll show you how to treat yourself to everything from pancakes, waffles, and muffins for breakfast to fried chicken, pizza, pasta, and enchiladas for dinner—over 300 easy-to-prepare recipes for your favorite comfort foods, all low-carb and in perfect sync with your commitment to good health. Staying on a low-carb plan for the long term has never been easier—or tastier!

CHAPTER 4

The 30-Day Low-Carb Diet Solution

Meal Plans

Now you're ready to eat! The meal plans presented here are intended to guide you through 30 days of low-carb correction and provide a wide variety of foods. In some cases, the choices may be foods you can't eat or don't like. That's okay. The plans are highly flexible. We've scaled them in such a way that you may interchange any breakfast for another one, any lunch for another lunch, any snack for another snack, and any dinner for another dinner. Or if you want to keep it extremely simple to follow—say if you don't cook, you're dining out, or you're on the road—just use the generic meal plan that follows to compose a simple meal. And don't forget that if you're in a rush you can always substitute a Power Shake* for any meal. Please note that an (*) beside an item indicates that the recipe appears in the book.

Although we haven't included them with each meal, you may have as much regular or decaf coffee, black or herbal tea, or still or sparkling water as you'd like with your meals and throughout the day—and if you'd like, a glass of wine or a light beer with a meal. Diet beverages that don't contain aspartame are also okay at any time.

Note, too, that we've tried to limit your kitchen work by such tricks as planning lunches from dinner leftovers on successive days.

Generic Ultra-Low Ultra-Easy Meal Plan

BREAKFAST Eggs, any style, with bacon, ham, sausage or fish, if desired

1 slice low-carb toast with butter

LUNCH Bacon Cheeseburger or grilled chicken breast *sans* bun

Salad greens with dressing

SNACK ½ small serving of fruit and/or dry-roasted nuts or cheese

DINNER Grilled/broiled steak, chicken, fish

½-to-1 cup green or colorful low-starch vegetable

Salad greens with real dressing

½ cup berries

The 30-Day Solution

Day 1

BREAKFAST Ham and cheese omelet

½ cup strawberries

1 slice low-carb toast with butter

LUNCH Tuna salad

1 cup lettuce with olive oil vinaigrette

SNACK 1 ounce dry-roasted nuts

DINNER Roasted Paprika Chicken*

1 serving Matilda's Green Beans*

1 serving Cukes and Onions*

Day 2

BREAKFAST   Power Shake*

LUNCH   Chicken Caesar Salad*

1 serving Orange and Strawberry Cup*

SNACK   1–2 ounces string cheese

DINNER   Grilled/Broiled Steak

1 serving Asparagus Parmesano*

1 sliced fresh tomato (or ½ cup canned)

1 serving Mini Chocolate Chip Cheesecake*

Day 3

BREAKFAST   Fruity Power Smoothie*

LUNCH   Tuna Salad Wrap*

Salad greens with good dressing

SNACK   1–2 ounces dry roasted nuts

DINNER   Kaye's Quiche*

1 serving Salad de Floret*

Salad greens with good dressing[1]

½ cup raspberries (a dollop of whipped cream, if desired)

Day 4

BREAKFAST   Yogurt Power Cup*

LUNCH   Cold roasted chicken

1 serving Salad de Floret*

SNACK   1 small tangerine

DINNER   Shrimp K-Bobs*

Salad greens with good dressing

1 serving Mini Chocolate Chip Cheesecake*

[1]All dressings should be "real"—made with good quality oils (page 38), real cream, sour cream, yogurt, or cheeses, but low in carbs. Commercial dressings should contain fewer than 2 grams carb per tablespoon. When you want to sweeten your own dressings, use Splenda or Stevia.

Day 5

BREAKFAST	Veggie Frittata*
	1 tomato, sliced (or ½ cup canned)
LUNCH	Chicken Salad-Stuffed Tomato*
	2–3 saltine crackers with butter (if desired)
SNACK	1–2 ounces dry-roasted nuts
DINNER	Broiled Salmon Steaks with Chive Butter*
	1 cup Sautéed Broccoli*
	Salad greens with good dressing
	½ cup berries (a dollop of whipped cream, if desired)

Day 6

BREAKFAST	Sausage and Egg Breakfast Burrito*
	½ tangerine
LUNCH	Grilled Salmon Caesar Salad*
	½ cup mixed fruit
SNACK	1–2 ounces hard cheese
DINNER	BBQ Chicken Wings* (or pieces)
	1 serving Homemade Coleslaw*
	Salad greens with good dressing
	1 serving Strawberry Cheesecake*

Day 7

BREAKFAST	Fruity Power Smoothie*
LUNCH	BBQ Chicken Wings*
	1 serving Coleslaw*
SNACK	1 ounce hard cheese and 1 ounce hard salami
DINNER	Stuffed Veal*
	Zucchini Medley*
	Green salad with good dressing
	1 serving Strawberry Cheesecake*

Day 8

BREAKFAST	Cheese Omelet*
	Sausage links
	1 serving Paleolithic Punch*
LUNCH	Lettuce-wrapped bacon double cheeseburger
	(or on a low-carb tortilla, low-carb bun)
	Green salad with good dressing
SNACK	½ apple with 2 tablespoons peanut butter
DINNER	Weight-Loss Chili*
	Salad greens with good dressing
	1 serving Strawberry Cheesecake*

Day 9

BREAKFAST	Eggs, any style
	4–6 spears steamed asparagus (with Blender Hollandaise*)
	½ cup strawberries
LUNCH	Weight-Loss Chili*
	Salad greens with good dressing
SNACK	1–2 ounces dry-roasted nuts
DINNER	Fish and Peppers*
	½ cup zucchini (sautéed in butter or olive oil)
	1 fresh tomato (or ½ cup canned)
	1 serving Mini Chocolate Chip Cheesecake*

Day 10

BREAKFAST	Eggs, any style
	Bacon
	1 slice low-carb toast with butter
LUNCH	Chicken Salad Wrap*
	½ fresh apple

SNACK ½ fresh apple with 2 tablespoons peanut butter

DINNER Easy Pork Tenderloin*

Sauteed Mushrooms*

Salad greens with good dressing

½ cup applesauce

Day 11

BREAKFAST Hardboiled Eggs and Bacon

1 Slice low-carb toast, buttered

½ cup strawberries

LUNCH Cold sliced pork Chef Salad*

SNACK 1 cup broccoli and cauliflower florets with good ranch dressing

DINNER Roast Pork Stir-fry*

Salad greens with a sesame oil vinaigrette

1 serving Orange-Strawberry Cup*

Day 12

BREAKFAST Power Shake*

LUNCH Tuna Salad Wrap*

Hardboiled egg

½ cup raspberries

DINNER Grilled Lamb Burgers*

1 serving Tangy Cabbage*

1 fresh tomato, wedged, with vinaigrette

Day 13

BREAKFAST Yogurt Power Cup*

LUNCH Grilled Lamb Burger Wrap*

(with diced tomato, lettuce, and Minted Yogurt Dressing*)

SNACK ½ cup grapes and 1–2 ounces hard cheese

DINNER	Grilled/broiled Steak
	1 serving Tangy Cabbage*
	1 fresh tomato, sliced, with vinaigrette
	½ cup grapes

Day 14

BREAKFAST	Breakfast Burrito with Cream Cheese*
LUNCH	Egg Salad Wrap*
	Salad greens with good dressing
	½ cup raspberries
SNACK	1–2 ounces dry-roasted nuts
DINNER	Skillet Chicken Italiano*
	Salad greens with vinaigrette
	1 serving Strawberry Cheesecake*

Day 15

BREAKFAST	Fruity Power Smoothie*
LUNCH	Hamburger patty
	Tomato and Mozzarella Salad*
	½ tangerine
SNACK	½ tangerine and 1 ounce dry-roasted nuts
DINNER	Broiled or sautéed shrimp
	1 serving Homestyle Tomato Soup*
	Salad greens with good dressing
	1 serving Strawberry Cheesecake*

Day 16

BREAKFAST	Power Shake*
LUNCH	Tuna Salad Wrap*
	½ orange
SNACK	½ orange with 1 ounce dry-roasted nuts
DINNER	Cinder's Lemon Chicken*

1 cup Sautéed Cauliflower*

1 fresh tomato, in wedges, with vinaigrette

1 serving Strawberry Cheesecake*

Day 17

BREAKFAST   Lighter-than-Air Pancakes* with butter

1 serving Mixed-Berry Syrup*

LUNCH   Cinder's Lemon Chicken*

1 serving Homestyle Tomato Soup*

SNACK   1 small tangerine

DINNER   Fish of your choice with lemon butter

1 serving Eggplant Milano*

1 serving Butter Lettuce Salad*

Day 18

BREAKFAST   Eggs, any style

Sausage

1 slice low-carb toast with butter and Strawberry
Preserves* (if desired)

LUNCH   Chicken Salad-Stuffed Tomato*

Salad greens with good dressing

½ cup raspberries

SNACK   1–2 ounces hard cheese

DINNER   Hobo Dinner Pork Chops*

1 fresh tomato (or ½ cup canned)

Salad greens with good dressing

1 serving Strawberry Cheesecake*

Day 19

BREAKFAST   Fruity Power Smoothie*

LUNCH   Chef Salad* with good dressing

SNACK   ½ cup grapes and 1–2 ounces hard cheese

DINNER   Beef K-Bobs*

Salad greens with good dressing

½ cup berries (dollop of whipped cream, if desired)

Day 20

BREAKFAST   Cottage cheese

½ cup berries

Crisp bacon

LUNCH   Chicken Salad-Stuffed Tomato*

2–3 saltine crackers with butter (if desired)

SNACK   1–2 ounces of deli meat and cheese and ½ cup grapes

DINNER   Grilled/broiled chicken breast

4 spears steamed asparagus with Blender
    Hollandaise*

1 serving Tomato and Mozzarella Salad*

1 serving Mini Chocolate Chip Cheesecake*

Day 21

BREAKFAST   Ham and Cheese Omelet*

1 slice low-carb toast, buttered

½ serving Paleolithic Punch*

LUNCH   Tuna Salad Wrap*

½ cup melon

SNACK   1–2 ounce dry-roasted nuts

DINNER   Roman-Style Chicken*

Salad greens with good dressing

1 serving Mini Chocolate Chip Cheesecake*

Day 22

BREAKFAST   Breakfast Burrito with Cream Cheese*

Sausage links

LUNCH   Chicken Caesar Salad*

2–3 saltine crackers with butter, if desired

SNACK   ½ cup grapes and 1–2 ounces string cheese

DINNER   Easy Pork Tenderloin*

½ cup green beans

Salad greens and tomato wedges with good dressing

Day 23

BREAKFAST   Yogurt Power Cup*

LUNCH   Roast pork tenderloin Wrap

Salad greens with good dressing

SNACK   ½ tangerine and 1–2 ounces hard cheese

DINNER   Halibut Jardinière*

1 serving Salad de Floret*

1 serving Mini Chocolate Chip Cheesecake*

Day 24

BREAKFAST   Eggs, any style, with bacon

1 slice low-carb toast, buttered

½ cup berries

LUNCH   Lettuce-wrapped bacon double cheeseburger

1 small orange

SNACK   1 serving Hot Chocolate*

1–2 ounces dry-roasted nuts

DINNER   Tabasco Chicken*

1 serving Herbed Brussels Sprouts

Salad greens with good dressing

½ cup berries (dollop of whipped cream, if desired)

Note: The final week of meal plans contains a slightly higher carbohydrate count per meal. They are to be used as you move toward maintenance. To use them in the corrective phase, simply eat half the specified amount of any food marked with a downward arrow.

Day 25

BREAKFAST   Eggs Benedict*
1 cup strawberries ↓

LUNCH   Tabasco Chicken* Wrap
1 fresh peach, sliced ↓

SNACK   ½ fresh peach, sliced and 1–2 ounces string cheese

DINNER   Broiled Salmon Steaks with Chive Butter*
Butter Lettuce Salad*
1 serving Tomato and Mozzarella Salad*
1 serving Mini Chocolate Chip Cheesecake*

Day 26

BREAKFAST   Power Shake*

LUNCH   Salmon Caesar Salad*
2–3 saltine crackers with butter, if desired
1 cup melon ↓

SNACK   1 small orange ↓ and 1–2 ounces hard cheese

DINNER   Easy Pork Tenderloin*
1 serving Skillet Ratatouille*
Salad greens with good dressing

Day 27

BREAKFAST   Eggs, any style
Sausage links

1 slice low-carb toast with butter and Strawberry
    Preserves* ↓

½ cup melon ↓

LUNCH   Pork Tenderloin* wrap

1 small peach ↓

Salad greens with good dressing

SNACK   1 small apple ↓ with 1–2 ounces Boursin cheese (or
    other herbed cream cheese)

DINNER   Rosemary Chicken*

1 serving Sadie Kendall's Mushroom Soup* ↓

Salad greens with good dressing

1 tomato, in wedges, with good dressing ↓

1 serving Strawberry Cheesecake*

Day 28

BREAKFAST Fruity Power Smoothie*

LUNCH   Chicken Salad Wrap*

1 tangerine ↓

SNACK   1 cup grapes ↓ with 1–2 ounces string cheese

DINNER   Grilled Lamb Burgers*

1 serving Italian Zucchini Bake* ↓

Salad greens with Minted Yogurt Dressing*

½ cup sliced peaches (dollop of whipped cream, if
    desired) ↓

Day 29

BREAKFAST 1 serving Lighter-than-Air Pancakes* with butter

1 serving Mixed-Berry Syrup*

Crisp bacon

1 cup melon ↓

LUNCH   Lamb Burger Wrap*

1 cup grapes ↓

Salad greens with good dressing

SNACK   1 small apple ↓ with 1–2 ounces hard cheese

DINNER   Grilled kielbasa, or Italian sausage

1 serving Tangy Cabbage*

1 serving Zucchini Medley* ↓

1 slice low-carb garlic toast (toasted with butter and a sprinkle of garlic powder) ↓

Day 30

BREAKFAST   Cheese Omelet*

Crisp bacon

2 servings Paleolithic Punch* ↓

LUNCH   Tuna Salad Wrap*

1 cup grapes ↓

SNACK   1 cup mixed melon cubes ↓ and 1–2 ounces beef jerky or deli meat

DINNER   1 serving Hobo Dinner Pork Chops* ↓ (reduce vegetables by half)

Salad greens with good dressing

½ cup raspberries (dollop of whipped cream, if desired)

1 glass champagne to celebrate completing your first 30 days of low-carb living!

Congratulations! You've now completed the first month on *The 30-Day Low-Carb Diet Solution.* If your main concern was lowering your cholesterol, triglycerides, blood sugar, or blood pressure, or if you had fewer than 15 to 20 pounds to lose, you've probably almost reached your goal. Now your job will be to maintain what you've worked to achieve—ongoing good health. If you had a significant amount of weight to lose or have not quite normalized your pressure or lipids, continue using the corrective level of *The 30-Day Low-Carb Diet Solution* until you near your goals. You can continue to use the meal plans for days 1 through 24 (or the scaled-down versions of days 25–30) or design your own meals using the appropriate Protein Servings List for your size and the Small Carbohydrate Servings List.

And Then What?

Once you've hit your targets in weight, blood pressure, or blood lipid readings, you should slowly begin to increase your carbohydrate intake, staying at the moderate level for a few weeks and then moving up to the large serving level for the long haul. The amount of carbohydrate intake you will tolerate and still maintain your correction will be specific to your own underlying metabolic sensitivities as well as your activity. The more active you are, the more carbohydrate you will tolerate without regaining weight or causing your blood pressure, blood sugar, or blood lipids to begin to rise again. These values should be your bellwether— if they begin to creep out of line, immediately focus on keeping your intake of carb-containing foods controlled until the numbers fall back to normal for you. You may even have to return to the corrective phase of the diet for a week or two to corral your metabolism now and again.

Be assured that by strictly following the principles of *The 30-Day Low-Carb Diet Solution* you will be able to reclaim and maintain your health, fitness, vigor, and stronger, leaner body, no matter what condition you're in.

Congratulations on your accomplishments so far. We'd love to hear about your success on the plan! You'll find our address in the Resources section on page 171.

To help you better visualize portion sizes, we've also included some actual-sized food illustrations in Appendix C on pages 174 and 175.

Protein Servings List
SMALL SERVING

Meats (includes beef, pork, lamb, poultry, game)	3 ounces
Fish (includes saltwater, freshwater, and shellfish)	3 ounces
Eggs	3 whole eggs or 2 eggs + 2 whites
Cottage Cheese (or other curd-style cheeses)*	¾ cup
Tofu*	4 ounces
Eggs and Bacon, Ham, Sausage, or Fish	2 eggs + 1 ounce meat or fish or 2 strips bacon or 1 link sausage
To add hard cheeses*	Substitute 1 ounce cheese for 1 egg or 1 ounce meat or fish
Protein Powder*	about 20 grams per serving

Protein Servings List
MEDIUM SERVING

Meats (includes beef, pork, lamb, poultry, game)	4 ounces
Fish (includes saltwater, freshwater, and shellfish)	4 ounces
Eggs	4 whole eggs or 2 eggs + 2 whites
Cottage Cheese (or other curd-style cheeses)*	1 cup
Tofu*	6 ounces
Eggs and Bacon, Ham, Sausage, or Fish	2 eggs + 2 whites + 1 ounce meat or fish or 2 strips bacon or 1 link sausage

*These combination foods contain both protein *and* carbohydrate. Please see the list on page 169 for their carbohydrate contents.

| To add hard cheeses* | Substitute 1 ounce cheese for 1 egg or 1 ounce meat or fish |
| Protein Powder* | about 27 grams per serving |

Protein Servings List
LARGE SERVING

Meats (includes beef, pork, lamb, poultry, game)	5 ounces
Fish (includes saltwater, freshwater, and shellfish)	5 ounces
Eggs	3 whole eggs + 4 whites
Cottage Cheese (or other curd-style cheeses)*	1¼ cups
Tofu*	7 ounces
Eggs and Bacon, Ham, Sausage, or Fish	4 eggs or 2 eggs + 2 whites and 1 ounce meat or fish or 2 strips bacon or 1 link sausage
To add hard cheeses*	Substitute 1 ounce cheese for 1 egg or 1 ounce meat or fish
Protein Powder*	about 34 grams per serving

Protein Servings List
EXTRA-LARGE SERVING

Meats (includes beef, pork, lamb, poultry, game)	6 ounces
Fish (includes saltwater, freshwater, and shellfish)	6 ounces
Eggs	3 whole eggs + 6 whites
Cottage Cheese (or other curd-style cheeses)*	1½ cups
Tofu*	8 ounces
Eggs and Bacon, Ham, Sausage, or Fish	3 eggs + 3 ounces meat or fish or 4 strips bacon or 3 links sausage

To add hard cheeses*	Substitute 1 ounce cheese for 1 egg or for 1 ounce meat or fish
Protein Powder*	about 40 grams per serving

Protein Servings List

EXTRA-EXTRA-LARGE SERVING

Meats (includes beef, pork, lamb, poultry, game)	8 ounces
Fish (includes saltwater, freshwater, and shellfish)	8 ounces
Eggs	4 whole eggs + 6 whites
Cottage Cheese (or other curd-style cheeses)*	2 cups
Tofu*	10 ounces
Eggs and Bacon, Ham, Sausage, or Fish	3 eggs + 4 ounces meat or fish or 6 strips bacon or 4 links sausage
To add hard cheeses*	Substitute 1 ounce cheese for 1 egg or for 1 ounce meat or fish
Protein Powder*	about 48 grams per serving

Carbohydrate Serving List

SMALL SERVING

During the corrective phase of your diet it's all-important to control your carb intake throughout the day. To construct your own meals at this earliest stage, you may choose two small carbohydrate servings at each meal or snack to stay within your carbohydrate limit. You might choose:

1 serving of fruit and 1 serving of a vegetable—or—

1 serving of fruit and 1 serving of bread/cereal/grain—or—

1 serving of vegetable and 1 serving of bread/cereal/grain—or—

2 servings of fruit —or—

2 servings of vegetable

We would encourage you not to take both your servings as bread/cereal/grain as a general rule, since this category of foods is in most cases nutritionally pretty empty.

Assume all whole fruits and vegetables to be of medium size, unless specified otherwise.

Fruits

¼ apple

¼ cup applesauce

2 apricots

½ avocado

½ cup blackberries

⅓ cup blueberries

½ cup cantaloupe

5 whole sweet cherries

¼ cup sour cherries (canned)

⅓ cup cranberries (raw)

2 teaspoons jellied cranberry sauce

½ cup black currants

¼ cup canned fruit cocktail

¼ grapefruit

¼ cup canned grapefruit

⅓ cup grapes

½ guava

½ cup honeydew melon

½ kiwi

½ orange

1 passionfruit

½ peach

⅓ cup canned peaches (in water)

¼ pear

¼ cup pineapple (raw)

½ plum

1 prune

½ cup raspberries

¾ cup strawberries

½ cup strawberries (frozen, unsweetened)

½ tangerine

½ cup watermelon

Vegetables

¼ artichoke (whole)

¼ cup artichoke hearts

1–2 cups arugula

10 spears asparagus (fresh)

1 cup canned asparagus

1 cup bamboo shoots

½ cup black soybeans

½ cup beets

2 cups broccoli (raw)

1 cup broccoli (cooked)

Vegetables (continued)

1 cup broccoli/cauliflower (frozen)

5 Brussels sprouts

1½ cups cabbage (raw)

1 cup cabbage (cooked)

1 medium carrot (raw)

½ cup carrots (cooked)

2 cups cauliflower (raw)

1½ cups cauliflower (cooked)

4 stalks celery (raw)

¾ cup celery (cooked)

¾ cup chard (cooked)

(unlimited) chives

⅓ cup homemade coleslaw

½ cucumber (raw)

¾ cup eggplant (cooked)

1–2 cups endive (raw)

¾ cup fennel (fresh)

3 cloves garlic

¼ cup sliced ginger (raw)

1 cup green beans (cooked)

1 cup green (spring) onions (raw)

½ cup greens (cooked)

½ cup kale (cooked)

¼ cup kelp (raw)

½ cup leeks (cooked)

(unlimited) lettuce

2 cups mushrooms (raw)

¾ cup mushrooms (cooked)

½ cup okra

½ cup onions (raw)

¼ cup onions (cooked)

(unlimited) parsley

⅓ cup green peas

½ cup chile peppers (canned)

1 whole chili pepper (raw)

½ sweet (bell) pepper (large, raw)

½ cup sweet (bell) pepper (cooked)

(unlimited) radicchio

(unlimited) radishes

½ cup rhubarb (cooked)

⅓ cup rutabaga (cooked)

½ cup sauerkraut

3 tablespoons shallots (raw)

(unlimited) spinach

½ cup spaghetti squash (cooked)

½ cup summer squash (cooked) (crookneck, scallop, zucchini)

⅓ cup winter squash (cooked) (acorn, butternut, hubbard)

2 tomatillos (raw)

1 tomato (raw)

½ cup tomato (canned)

1 cup turnips (boiled)

¼ cup water chestnuts (canned)

5 whole water chestnuts (canned)

½ cup wax beans

Bread, Cereal, and Grains

1 slice bread (commercial low-carb)

2–4 saltine crackers (commercial fat-free[2])

10 oyster crackers

1 Triscuit

2 Wasa crisp bread

2 Melba toast

8 Cheese nips

½ rice cake

⅛ cup rice

1 La Tortilla Factory low-carb tortilla[1]

Carbohydrate Serving List

MODERATE SERVING

As you approach your goal weight and/or target values for blood pressure, blood sugar, and blood lipids, you can begin to increase the amount of carbohydrate you're eating. As a guideline for constructing your own slightly higher-carb meals, you may choose two medium carbohydrate servings at each meal or snack. If you see your weight begin to sneak up again, drop back to the small level for a bit longer. A meal in the medium-carb range might include:

1 serving of fruit and 1 serving of a vegetable—or—

1 serving of fruit and 1 serving of bread/cereal/grain—or—

1 serving of vegetable and 1 serving of bread/cereal/grain—or—

2 fruit servings of fruit—or—

2 servings of vegetable

We would not encourage you to take both your servings as bread/cereal/grain as a general rule, since this category of foods is in most cases nutritionally pretty empty.

---

[1]Available in many stores. Also, see Resources for where you can obtain La Tortilla Factory tortillas by mail.

[2]Be aware that virtually all commercially baked goods contain *trans*fats, which have been shown to be a health hazard. Where possible, buy fat-free baked goods to avoid these bad fats, or make your own baked goods using the recipes in *The Low-Carb Comfort Food Cookbook*.

Assume all whole fruits or vegetables to be of medium size, unless specified otherwise.

Fruits

½ apple

½ cup applesauce

3 apricots (raw)

8 apricot halves (canned)

1 avocado

½ banana (small)

¾ cup blackberries

½ cup blueberries

¾ cup cantaloupe

10 whole sweet cherries

½ cup sour cherries (canned)

¾ cup cranberries (raw)

1 tbsp. jellied cranberry sauce

¾ cup black currants

1 date (whole)

1 fig

½ cup fruit cocktail (in water)

½ grapefruit (fresh)

⅓ cup canned grapefruit

½ cup grapes

1 guava

½ cup honeydew melon

1 kiwi

⅓ cup mandarin orange (in water)

¼ cup mango

½ nectarine

¾ orange

¼ papaya

2 passionfruit

1 peach

½ cup canned peaches (in water)

1 peach half (dried)

½ pear

½ pear, Asian

¼ cup pineapple

1 persimmon

1 plum

¼ pomegranate

2 prunes

½ quince

1 cup raspberries

1 cup strawberries (fresh)

¾ cup strawberries (frozen, unsweetened)

1 tangerine (medium)

¾ cup watermelon

Vegetables

1 cup alfalfa sprouts

½ artichoke (whole)

½ cup artichoke hearts

(unlimited) arugula

20 spears asparagus (fresh)

1½ cups canned asparagus

2 cups bamboo shoots

⅓ cup beans, dried (cooked)

¾ cup beets (boiled)

¼ cup beets, pickled (canned)

1 cup black soybeans

⅓ cup black eyed peas or cow-peas (canned)

4 cups broccoli (raw)

2 cups broccoli (cooked)

1½ cups broccoli and carrots (frozen)

2 cups broccoli and cauliflower (frozen)

10 Brussels sprouts (fresh)

⅓ cup butter beans (canned)

3 cups cabbage (raw)

2 cups cabbage (cooked)

2 carrots (raw)

¾ cup carrots (cooked)

4 cups cauliflower (raw)

2 cups cauliflower (cooked)

(unlimited) stalks celery (raw)

1½ cups celery (cooked)

1 cup chard (cooked)

¼ cup chickpeas or garbanzo beans (cooked)

(unlimited) chives

½ cup homemade coleslaw

¼ cup corn (cooked)

1 cucumber (raw)

1 cup eggplant (cooked)

4 cups endive (raw)

1 cup fennel (fresh)

(unlimited) cloves garlic

½ cup sliced ginger (raw)

1½ cups green beans (cooked)

2 cups green (spring) onions (raw)

1½ cups greens, beet, collard, turnip, mustard (cooked)

1 cup kale (cooked)

½ cup kelp (raw)

1 cup leeks (cooked)

(unlimited) lettuce

(unlimited) mushrooms (raw)

2 cups mushrooms (cooked)

¾ cup okra

¾ cup onions (raw)

½ cup onions (cooked)

(unlimited) parsley

½ cup green peas

1 cup chile peppers (canned)

2 whole chili peppers (raw)

1 sweet (bell) pepper (small, raw)

1½ cups sweet (bell) pepper (cooked)

(unlimited) radicchio

(unlimited) radishes

1 cup rhubarb (cooked)

½ cup rutabaga (cooked)

¾ cup sauerkraut

⅓ cup shallots (raw)

(unlimited) spinach

1 cup spaghetti squash (cooked)

1 cup summer squash (cooked—crookneck, scallop, zucchini)

Vegetables (continued)

⅔ cup winter squash (cooked)
(acorn, butternut, hubbard)

5 tomatillos (medium, raw)

2 tomatoes (medium, raw)

1 cup tomato (canned)

¼ cup sundried tomato

1 cup turnips (cooked)

½ cup water chestnuts (canned)
or 10 whole water chestnuts
(canned)

1 cup wax beans

¼ cup yams (cooked)

Bread, Cereal, and Grains

1 small biscuit or roll
(¾ ounce)

1½ slices bread (commercial
low-carb)

4 saltine crackers (commercial
fat-free)

20 oyster crackers (commercial
fat-free)

½ hamburger or hot dog bun
(commercial fat-free)

3 Triscuits

5 Wasa crisp bread

4 Melba toast

15 Cheese nips

½ small pita pocket

1 rice cake

¼ cup rice

2 La Tortilla Factory low-carb
tortillas[3]

1 taco shell (commercial)

Carbohydrate Serving List

LARGE SERVING

During the maintenance phase of your diet, you may pretty freely choose to eat from any of the serving lists in whatever combination suits you. Remember that the total carbohydrate content of a meal or snack will be the sum of all the fruit, vegetables, breads, cereals, grains, nuts, and dairy products it contains. For a simple guide to constructing your own meals, begin by choosing two large carbohy-

---

[3]Available in many stores. Also, see Resources for where you can obtain La Tortilla Factory tortillas by mail.

drate servings at each meal or snack and see how you do, increasing your carb intake from these good foods as you feel comfortable. Remember that if your weight begins to climb or your blood pressure, blood sugar, or blood lipids begin to rise, you must cut back again on the amount of carbohydrate that you're eating. Drop back to the strict definition of a large serving first. If necessary, go back to the medium or even to the small level for a few days and recover your weight, pressure, or return blood test values to normal before advancing again.

As you enter maintenance, begin by eating two large servings of carb at each meal or snack. This could include:

1 serving of fruit and 1 serving of a vegetable—or—

1 serving of fruit and 1 serving of bread/cereal/grain—or—

1 serving of vegetable and 1 serving of bread/cereal/grain—or—

2 servings of fruit—or—

2 servings of vegetable

We would not encourage you to take both your servings as bread/cereal/grain as a general rule, since this category of foods is in most cases nutritionally pretty empty.

Assume all whole fruits or vegetables to be of medium size, unless specified otherwise.

Fruits

¾ apple	¾ cup blueberries
¾ cup applesauce	1 cup cantaloupe
4 apricots (raw)	15 whole sweet cherries
12 apricot halves (canned)	¾ cup sour cherries (canned)
2 avocado	1 cup cranberries (raw)
½ banana (medium)	2 tbsp. jellied cranberry sauce
1¼ cups blackberries	1 cup black currants

Fruits (continued)

2 dates (whole)

1½ figs

¾ cup fruit cocktail (in water)

¾ grapefruit (fresh)

⅔ cup canned grapefruit

1 cup grapes

1½ guavas

1 cup honeydew melon

1½ kiwis

½ cup mandarin orange (in water)

½ cup mango

1 nectarine

1 orange

½ papaya

3 passionfruits

1½ peaches

1 cup canned peaches (in water)

1½ peach halves (dried)

¾ pear

1 pear, Asian

¾ cup pineapple

1½ persimmons

1½ plums

½ pomegranate

3 prunes

1 quince

1¾ cups raspberries

2 cups strawberries (fresh)

1½ cups strawberries (frozen, unsweetened)

1½ tangerines (medium)

1 cup watermelon

Vegetables

(unlimited) alfalfa sprouts

1 artichoke (whole)

¾ cup artichoke hearts

(unlimited) arugula

25 spears asparagus (fresh)

2 cups canned asparagus

3 cups bamboo shoots

½ cup beans, dried (cooked)

1 cup beets (boiled)

⅓ cup beets, pickled (canned)

1½ cups black soybeans

½ cup black eyed peas or cow-peas (canned)

(unlimited) broccoli (raw)

3 cups broccoli (cooked)

2 cups broccoli & carrots (frozen)

2½ cups broccoli & cauliflower (frozen)

15 Brussels sprouts (fresh)

½ cup butter beans (canned)

(unlimited) cabbage (raw)

3 cups cabbage (cooked)

3 carrots (raw)

1 cup carrots (cooked)

5 cups cauliflower (raw)

3 cups cauliflower (cooked)

(unlimited) stalks celery (raw)

2 cups celery (cooked)

1 cup chard (cooked)

⅓ cup chickpeas or garbanzo beans (cooked)

(unlimited) chives

1 cup homemade coleslaw

⅓ cup corn (cooked)

2 cucumbers (raw)

2 cups eggplant (cooked)

(unlimited) endive (raw)

2 cups fennel (fresh)

(unlimited) cloves garlic

¾ cup sliced ginger (raw)

2 cups green beans (cooked)

(unlimited) green (spring) onions (raw)

2 cups greens, beet, collard, turnip, mustard (cooked)

2 cups kale (cooked)

⅔ cup kelp (raw)

1½ cups leeks (cooked)

(unlimited) lettuce

(unlimited) mushrooms (raw)

3 cups mushrooms (cooked)

1 cup okra

¾ cup onions (raw)

½ cup onions (cooked)

(unlimited) parsley

¾ cup green peas

1¾ cups chile peppers (canned)

3 whole chili peppers (raw)

1 sweet (bell) pepper (large, raw)

2 cups sweet (bell) pepper (cooked)

¼ potato, baked with skin

⅓ cup potato, mashed

½ cup pumpkin

(unlimited) radicchio

(unlimited) radishes

1½ cups rhubarb (cooked)

1 cup rutabaga (cooked)

1 cup sauerkraut

(unlimited) shallots (raw)

(unlimited) spinach

1½ cups spaghetti squash (cooked)

3 cups summer squash (cooked) (crookneck, scallop, zucchini)

1 cup winter squash (cooked) (acorn, butternut, hubbard)

7 tomatillos (medium, raw)

3 tomatoes (medium, raw)

1½ cups tomato (canned)

½ cup sundried tomato

3 cups turnips (cooked)

¾ cup water chestnuts (canned)

15 whole water chestnuts (canned)

Vegetables (continued)

1½ cups wax beans

⅓ cup yams (cooked)

Bread/Cereal/Grain

½ bagel (medium)

1 medium biscuit or roll (1 ounce)

2 slices bread (commercial low-carb)

6 saltine crackers (commercial fat-free)[4]

25 oyster crackers (commercial fat-free)

⅓ cup couscous (cooked)

½ English muffin (commercial fat-free)

1 hamburger or hot dog bun (commercial fat-free)

5 Triscuits

7 Wasa crisp bread

6 Melba toast

25 cheese nips

1 small pita pocket

2 rice cakes

⅓ cup rice

3 La Tortilla Factory low-carb tortillas[5]

1 fajita wrap (small, commercial)

2 taco shells (commercial)

1 waffle (small, frozen, commercial)

---

[4]Be aware that virtually all commercially baked goods contain *trans*fats, which have been shown to be a health hazard. Where possible, buy fat-free baked goods to avoid these bad fats, or make your own baked goods using the recipes in *The Low-Carb Comfort Food Cookbook*.
[5]Available in many stores. Also, see Resources for where you can obtain La Tortilla Factory tortillas by mail.

CHAPTER 5

Recipes

Egg Dishes and Breakfast Foods

Veggie Frittata

NUMBER OF SERVINGS: 2

NUTRITIONAL VALUES PER SERVING: 2.0 grams of carb, 21.5 grams of protein

6	whole eggs (whites and yolks together)
1	ounce hard cheese of your choice, grated
¼	red pepper, chopped
1	cup fresh spinach, chopped
½	cup fresh mushrooms, chopped
1 to 2	tablespoons unsalted butter
	salt and pepper, to taste

Beat eggs together in a bowl.

Melt butter in heavy, oven-safe skillet.

Pour beaten eggs into skillet over high heat.

Stir mixture gently to allow eggs to set.

When eggs are nearly halfway set, add vegetables to egg mixture.

Top with grated cheese.

Set oven to broil.

Place skillet in the oven and leave oven door slightly open.

When cheese bubbles, frittata is done—to be sure, you can cut with a knife to make sure mixture has solidified all the way through.

Breakfast Extravaganza

NUMBER OF SERVINGS: 4

NUTRITIONAL VALUES PER SERVING: 5.2 grams of carb, 12.9 grams of protein

2	tablespoons butter
½	white onion, chopped
1	teaspoon garlic, minced
½	eggplant, peeled and diced
¼	cup fresh bell pepper, chopped
¼	cup fresh mushrooms, chopped
8	eggs
1	teaspoon black pepper
1	teaspoon Herbes de Provence
1	teaspoon salt

Melt butter in a large skillet.

Sauté onion and garlic until transparent.

Add eggplant, bell pepper, and mushrooms.

Sauté all until just done (cooked, but still crunchy).

In a mixing bowl, beat eggs until frothy.

Beat in black pepper, herbs and salt.

Pour egg mixture into skillet with sautéed vegetables.

Mix ingredients gently with a large spoon until eggs are cooked.

Casserole Egg-stravaganza

NUMBER OF SERVINGS: 6

NUTRITIONAL VALUES PER SERVING: 1.6 grams of carb, 18.7 grams of protein

6   pieces raw bacon
12   eggs
4   ounces Monterey Jack cheese
     salt, pepper, and Herbes de Provence, to taste

Spray 2-quart casserole dish with no-stick cooking spray or grease lightly with coconut oil.

Dice bacon into the casserole dish.

Microwave on high 2 to 3 minutes, until done.

Beat the eggs in a mixing bowl.

Grate Monterey Jack cheese into the eggs.

Add salt, pepper, and herbs.

Pour egg mixture into the casserole dish with the bacon already in it.

Cover and microwave on high for 3 minutes.

Stir and continue microwaving for 2 more minutes on high.

Check for doneness.

Continue microwaving on high, 30 seconds at a time, stirring between each time, until done.

Swiss Egg Casserole

NUMBER OF SERVINGS: 2

NUTRITIONAL VALUES PER SERVING: 4.5 grams of carb, 29.1 grams of protein

4	1-ounce slices Swiss cheese
4	eggs
⅛	teaspoon nutmeg
⅛	teaspoon caraway seeds
½	teaspoon Krazy Mixed-up Salt or seasoned salt
2	tablespoons butter
¼	cup heavy cream
	dash pepper

Preheat oven to 400°.

Coat a baking dish with no-stick cooking spray or grease lightly with coconut oil.

Line the bottom of the pan with 2 1-ounce slices of Swiss cheese.

Beat eggs in a separate bowl.

Add nutmeg, caraway seeds, and Krazy Mixed-up Salt or seasoned salt.

Pour mixture into the baking dish.

Top with the remaining Swiss cheese.

Dot with butter.

Pour on heavy cream.

Sprinkle on pepper.

Bake at 400° for 15 minutes.

Kaye's Quiche

NUMBER OF SERVINGS: 6

NUTRITIONAL VALUES PER SERVING: 3.1 grams of carb, 14.6 grams of protein

1	tablespoon butter
3	tablespoons raw onion, minced
4	slices crisp bacon
5	eggs
1	10-ounce package frozen spinach, chopped
½	cup cheese, grated

Thaw spinach and drain excess water ahead of time.

Coat a quiche pan with no-stick cooking spray or coconut oil.

In a skillet, melt butter.

Sauté onion until clear; set aside.

Cook bacon until crisp; crumble.

In a mixing bowl, beat the eggs.

Add onion, bacon, spinach, and cheese.

Pour mixture into the quiche pan.

Bake at 350° for 30 to 35 minutes.

Egg Salad

NUMBER OF SERVINGS: 4 (as wraps)

NUTRITIONAL VALUES PER SERVING: 1.9 grams of carb, 12.4 grams of protein

8   eggs
2   tablespoons black olives, chopped
1   teaspoon onion, minced
½   teaspoon garlic powder
1   tablespoon dill pickle, chopped
2   tablespoons Homemade Mayonnaise*, or to taste
1   tablespoon Dijon-style mustard

Hard-boil eggs and cool quickly under running water.

Peel and chop the eggs.

Add black olives, onion, garlic powder, dill pickle, mayonnaise, and mustard.

Mix well.

Delightfully Devilish Eggs

NUMBER OF SERVINGS: 6

NUTRITIONAL VALUES PER SERVING: 0.5 gram of carb, 4.4 grams of protein

6　large eggs
¼　cup salmon, drained and boned
¼　cup cream cheese, softened
¼　teaspoon garlic powder
　　salt and pepper, to taste
　　caviar, a sprinkle *or*
　　capers, a few *or*
1　black olive (if desired), sliced

Hard-boil the eggs ahead of time.

Peel then slice the eggs in halves.

Set whites aside.

Place egg yolks in a separate bowl.

In the bowl, mash the yolks with a fork.

Add salmon, cream cheese, garlic powder, salt, and pepper.

Beat the mixture until smooth.

Stuff mixture into the egg white halves.

Garnish with caviar, capers or olives.

Sausage and Egg Breakfast Burrito

NUMBER OF SERVINGS: 1

NUTRITIONAL VALUES PER SERVING: 10.7 grams of carb, 25 grams of protein

2   large eggs, beaten
1   ounce sausage
½   teaspoon black pepper
1   large tortilla, La Tortilla Factory, low-carb*
2   tablespoons commercial salsa (if desired)

Crumble sausage into a skillet and fry until done. Add the pepper to the eggs, the eggs to the skillet, and scramble with the sausage.

Warm tortilla on hot griddle or in microwave for 20 to 30 seconds on high.

Place the scrambled eggs and sausage in the center, fold both sides in, and roll up.

Top with salsa, if desired.

*These are available from the La Tortilla Factory only. See Resources for 1-800 number where you can order.

Breakfast Burrito with Cream Cheese

NUMBER OF SERVINGS: 1

NUTRITIONAL VALUES PER SERVING: 10.0 grams of carb, 16.0 grams of protein

- ½   cup cottage cheese
- 1   ounce cream cheese
- 3 or 4 fresh strawberries
- 1   large tortilla, La Tortilla Factory, low-carb*

The night before:

Blend cottage cheese, cream cheese, and strawberries in blender until creamy.

Place mixture in a strainer, lined with a coffee filter and allow to drain in the refrigerator overnight.

To serve:

Warm tortilla on a hot griddle for 15 seconds each side.

Place cheese and fruit mixture in the center of warmed tortilla.

Roll and serve seam side down.

*These are available from the La Tortilla Factory only. See Resources for 1-800 number where you can order.

Lighter-than-Air Pancakes

NUMBER OF SERVINGS: 2

NUTRITIONAL VALUES PER SERVING: 10.5 grams of carb, 14.0 grams of protein

2	extra-large eggs
⅓	cup cottage cheese
2	tablespoons cream cheese, softened
1	packet Splenda
3	tablespoons almond meal*
1	tablespoon whey protein powder*
1	teaspoon baking powder
	pinch baking soda

Whip the eggs in a food processor or by hand until frothy.

Add the cheeses and beat until smooth.

Add artificial sweetener.

Add the rest of the ingredients and pulse to blend.

Gently scrape the batter into a small bowl.

Heat a no-stick skillet or griddle with a little butter as needed.

When griddle is hot, spoon the batter onto it.

Cook over medium heat until edges are set and large bubbles appear across the surface, about 1 minute.

Carefully flip and cook for half as long as on the first side or until golden.

Serve with a drizzle of dietetic or Mixed-Berry Syrup*.

*Almond meal and whey protein powders are available at most health food stores or at www.vitamincottage.com.

Power Shake

NUMBER OF SERVINGS: 1

NUTRITIONAL VALUES PER SERVING: usually 3 to 8 grams of carb, depending on
the protein powder used, protein value dependent on the number of
scoops of powder used

> Protein Powder*, any flavor
1 ounce heavy cream
1 packet Splenda (if desired)
8 ounces cold water or SoBe Lean†
1 cup ice

Place all ingredients into a blender and blend until thick and
smooth.

You can substitute any non-caloric beverage for the water or SoBe
Lean, but avoid those sweetened with aspartame. Good choices
include: herbal fruit teas, Tazo iced teas, and Diet RC. Also, be care-
ful to secure the blender top well if you select a carbonated beverage.

---

*Select a protein powder containing fewer than 3 grams of carbohydrate per scoop. Use
enough scoops to meet your protein serving requirement.
†You can find SoBe Lean, a diet beverage sweetened with sucralose, at many grocery stores
and discount chains. Be sure to select the Lean, as the other SoBe formulations have a significant sugar load.

Yogurt Power Cup

NUMBER OF SERVINGS: 1

NUTRITIONAL VALUES PER SERVING: 7.8 grams of carb plus the amount in each scoop of protein powder, 5.6 grams of protein plus the amount in each scoop of protein powder

½   cup plain yogurt (unsweetened, no added fruit or flavor)
    Protein powder*
⅛   cup pecans, chopped
1   packet Splenda or Stevia

Mix all ingredients together and enjoy.

As you progress through your plan and can tolerate a greater number of carbs, you can use the whole 8-ounce container of plain yogurt in this recipe if you choose.

---

*Select a protein powder containing fewer than 3 grams of carbohydrate per scoop. Use enough scoops to meet your protein serving requirement.

Paleolithic Punch*

NUMBER OF SERVINGS: 2

NUTRITIONAL VALUES PER SERVING: 7.9 grams of carb, 0.7 gram of protein

1½ cups frozen mixed berries (unsweetened)
½ to 1 cup water
1   packet Splenda (optional)

Place all ingredients into a heavy-duty blender and process until smooth and slushy. Begin with ½ cup water and add more water to thin, if necessary.

*From *The Protein Power LifePlan,* Michael R. Eades, M.D. and Mary Dan Eades, M.D.

Soups and Salads

Tomato and Mozzarella Salad

NUMBER OF SERVINGS: 1

NUTRITIONAL VALUES PER SERVING: 5.0 grams of carb, 11.0 grams of protein

- 1 medium ripe, red tomato
- 2 ounces fresh Buffalo mozzarella, sliced in ¼-inch slices
- 2 fresh basil leaves, cut up
- 1 to 2 tablespoons extra-virgin olive oil
- 1 teaspoon balsamic vinegar
  salt and pepper, to taste

Slice tomato into ¼-inch slices.

Layer tomato slices, then mozzarella slices, and so on.

Top with basil leaves.

Mix olive oil and vinegar and drizzle over salad.

Add salt and pepper to taste.

Homemade Coleslaw

NUMBER OF SERVINGS: 8

NUTRITIONAL VALUES PER SERVING: 5.3 grams of carb, 1.8 grams of protein

1   head cabbage, finely shredded
1   medium carrot, finely shredded
1   cup Homemade Mayonnaise*
¼   cup champagne (or white) vinegar
4   packets Splenda
½   teaspoon garlic powder
½   teaspoon celery seed
½   teaspoon each, salt and pepper

In a large bowl, thoroughly mix the mayonnaise, vinegar, Splenda, and spices to make a smooth, creamy dressing. Add the shredded cabbage and carrots and toss to completely coat. Cover and refrigerate.

Caesar Salad

NUMBER OF SERVINGS: 2

NUTRITIONAL VALUES PER SERVING: 2.9 grams of carb, 9.6 grams of protein

- 2 cups romaine lettuce, torn
- 3 tablespoons healthy commercial Caesar Dressing
- 4 anchovy fillets, if desired
- 1 tablespoon Parmesan cheese, freshly grated, if possible

Toss lettuce with dressing in a large bowl. Divide greens between two serving plates, top each serving with 2 anchovy fillets, and ½ the grated cheese.

Variation: Add leftover grilled, roasted, or canned chicken to make a Chicken Caesar or grilled, poached, or canned salmon for a Salmon Caesar to increase the protein about 7 grams per ounce of chicken or fish used.

Butter Lettuce Salad

NUMBER OF SERVINGS: 3 to 4

NUTRITIONAL VALUES PER SERVING: 5.7 grams of carb, 4.5 grams of protein

    1   medium head butter lettuce
    1   small can mandarin orange slices in water, drained
    ½   cup large walnut pieces
    ¼   cup olive or walnut oil
    1   tablespoon wine vinegar
    1   packet Splenda
    ½   teaspoon salt
    ½   teaspoon ground pepper

Wash, dry, and tear lettuce.

Chill in a cotton kitchen towel for several hours in refrigerator.

At serving time, place chilled greens into salad bowl.

Add mandarin orange slices and walnuts.

Toss with dressing (below) to coat well.

Dressing:

In a small bowl, mix oil, wine vinegar, sweetener, salt, and pepper.

Salad de Floret

NUMBER OF SERVINGS: 4 to 6

NUTRITIONAL VALUES PER SERVING: 7.2 grams of carb, 6.3 grams of protein

2	cups cauliflower
2	cups broccoli
¾	cup buttermilk
½	cup cottage cheese
1½	teaspoons dillweed, dried
½	teaspoon black pepper
1	teaspoon soy sauce

Wash and break florets from cauliflower and broccoli.

Place into large bowl and set aside.

In a blender or food processor, blend buttermilk, cottage cheese, dillweed, pepper, and soy sauce until smooth.

Pour dressing over florets and toss well.

Sesame Tofu Salad

NUMBER OF SERVINGS: 1

NUTRITIONAL VALUES PER SERVING: 5.0 grams of carb for 4 ounces, 8.0 grams of carb for 6 ounces, 19.0 grams of protein for 4 ounces, 28.0 grams of protein for 6 ounces

       2   cups mixed lettuce
       3   tablespoons olive oil vinaigrette
       4 to 6 ounces Sesame-seed Tofu*, baked, sliced in strips
       ½   avocado, sliced
       1   teaspoon sesame seeds
           salt and pepper, to taste

Dress lettuce lightly with 2 tablespoons olive oil vinaigrette.

Place lettuce leaves on a plate.

Arrange tofu and avocado slices on top.

Sprinkle with sesame seeds and remaining vinaigrette.

Add salt and pepper to taste.

*Available from the WhiteWave Company at most stores.

Chef's Salad

NUMBER OF SERVINGS: 1

NUTRITIONAL VALUES PER SERVING: 11.7 grams of carb, 21.1 grams of protein

1	cup iceberg lettuce
1	cup loose leaf lettuce
1	hard-boiled egg, sliced
¼	cup carrots, shredded
¼	cup green onion, chopped
⅓	cucumber, peeled and sliced
½	tomato, cut in wedges
1	ounce ham, diced or julienne
1	ounce hard cheese, shredded
	your favorite good quality dressing
	pepper, fresh-ground

Wash and tear iceberg lettuce and leaf lettuce.

Add egg, carrots, green onion, cucumber, tomato, ham, and cheese.

Top with your favorite dressing and fresh-ground pepper.

Avgolemono
(Greek Egg-and-Lemon Soup)

NUMBER OF SERVINGS: 6 to 8

NUTRITIONAL VALUES PER SERVING: 1.1 grams of carb, 4.5 grams of protein

2	10-ounce cans condensed chicken broth
1½	cups water
4	eggs
¼	cup lemon juice
1	lemon, sliced for garnish

In a saucepan, mix chicken broth and water, then heat to boiling. Reduce heat to very low.

In a separate bowl, beat eggs until foamy.

Beat in lemon juice.

Whisking constantly, slowly add a little hot broth to egg-and-lemon mixture.

Pour the egg-and-lemon mixture into the pan of broth, and cook over low heat, stirring constantly until thickened.

Pour into serving bowls, garnish with lemon slices.

Variation: Egg Drop Soup   Omit the lemon juice and lemon slice garnish. Substitute 1 teaspoon rice vinegar, ½ teaspoon black pepper, and garnish with 1 tablespoon chopped green onion.

Homestyle Tomato Soup

NUMBER OF SERVINGS: 4

NUTRITIONAL VALUES PER SERVING: 8.8 grams of carb, 4.4 grams of protein

⅛ cup olive oil
1   medium onion, thinly sliced
2   large garlic cloves, crushed
1   14½-ounce can tomatoes, diced
2   cans beef broth
¼   cup fresh parsley, chopped
½   teaspoon black pepper
1   teaspoon basil, dried

In a large saucepan, heat olive oil.

Sauté onion, garlic, and tomatoes.

Add beef bouillon or broth, parsley, black pepper, and basil.

Simmer for 30 minutes.

Sadie Kendall's Mushroom Soup

NUMBER OF SERVINGS: 4

NUTRITIONAL VALUES PER SERVING: 5.7 grams of carb, 4.7 grams of protein

1	tablespoon unsalted butter
2	tablespoons shallots (or onion), minced
1	pound fresh, firm mushrooms, coarsely chopped
¼	teaspoon thyme, dried
½	bay leaf
1	teaspoon salt
½	teaspoon fresh-ground black pepper
1½	cups chicken stock
1	cup crème fraîche

In a heavy saucepan, melt butter.

Sauté shallots (or onion).

Add mushrooms, thyme, and bay leaf.

Sauté until mushrooms release their liquid.

Add salt, pepper, and the chicken stock.

Simmer for 10 minutes.

Add 1 cup crème fraîche.

Simmer 2 minutes more.

Adjust seasonings to taste and serve warm.

Wraps

You can create an endless variety of delicious wraps using La Tortilla Factory's low-carb tortillas for a carb cost of 3 to 6 grams, depending on which wrap you choose[1].

Directions: Warm the tortilla on a hot griddle or in the microwave, according to package directions.

Place shredded lettuce or lettuce leaves, some diced tomato or avocado, and your choice of Homemade Mayonnaise*, mustard, dill relish, Minted Yogurt Dressing*, Mr. Ron's Barbecue Sauce* (or whatever low-carb condiment seems to go best with your wrap) onto the warm tortilla. Add slices of grilled chicken, steak, or fish, deli meats, cheeses, hamburger, lamb burger, veggie burgers, baked tofu, barbecued beef, pork, or chicken, egg salad, tuna salad, chicken salad, or shrimp salad in the center. The choices are endless. Fold the sides toward the middle, then roll the wrap securely around its contents.

---

[1] See Resources for where to order low-carb tortillas by mail. Or you can also make your own low-carb tortillas using the recipe from *The Low-Carb Comfort Food Cookbook,* available wherever books are sold.

Meat, Fish, and Fowl Dishes

Grilled Lamb Burgers

NUMBER OF SERVINGS: 4 (quarter-pounders)

NUTRITIONAL VALUES PER SERVING: 0 grams of carb, 28.0 grams of protein

- 1   pound lamb, ground
- 1   tablespoon parsley, finely chopped
- 1   tablespoon onion, finely chopped
- 1   garlic clove, chopped
- 1   teaspoon each, salt and pepper

Mix all ingredients.

Form into 4 patties.

Grill 4 to 5 minutes each side and serve.

Beef K-Bobs

NUMBER OF SERVINGS: 4

NUTRITIONAL VALUES PER SERVING: 12.1 grams of carb, 19.7 grams of protein

16   1-inch steak cubes
16   fresh mushrooms, whole
4   small onions
4   small bell peppers
     olive oil, for brushing
     black pepper, to taste

Tenderize and season the cubes of steak.

Wash mushrooms.

Peel and quarter onions.

Seed and cut bell peppers into 1-inch squares.

On 4 or 5 wooden or metal skewers, arrange meat, pepper, onion, and mushrooms in repeating pattern until the skewer is full.

Brush all with olive oil.

Sprinkle with ground black pepper.

Grill over medium- to red-hot coals for 4 minutes a side or until done.

Weight-Loss Chili

NUMBER OF SERVINGS: 4

NUTRITIONAL VALUES PER SERVING: 6.1 grams of carb, 20.9 grams of protein

¼   cup onion, chopped
¼   cup bell pepper, diced
¼   cup mushrooms, sliced or chopped
1   pound lean ground beef
1   small can tomatoes, sliced or whole (if whole, cut into pieces)
2   tablespoons chili powder (more or less to taste)
     salt

Spray a skillet with no-stick cooking spray or grease lightly with coconut oil.

Quickly sauté onion and bell pepper, then add and sauté mushrooms. Set aside.

Brown ground beef and drain fat.

In a deep saucepan or stockpot, combine browned beef, onion, mushrooms, pepper, tomatoes, and enough water to achieve desired thickness.

Blend in chili powder and salt to taste.

Simmer about 30 minutes.

Easy Beef or Pork Tenderloin

NUMBER OF SERVINGS: 6 to 8

NUTRITIONAL VALUES PER SERVING: 1.4 grams of carb, 22.0 grams of protein

1	tablespoon salt
1	tablespoon black pepper
2	teaspoons garlic powder
2	pounds tenderloin (beef or pork)

Preheat oven to 500°

Spray a baking dish with no-stick cooking spray or grease lightly with coconut oil.

On a piece of waxed paper, mix salt, pepper, and garlic powder.

Roll tenderloin in spices to coat.

Place loin in baking dish and place uncovered in hot oven.

Beef loin: Turn oven off immediately.

Pork loin: Leave oven on approximately 10 minutes, then turn off.

Do not open oven door for 4 hours or more. The residual heat from the oven will cook the loin to perfection without drying it out.

Slice and reheat gently for 30 seconds to one minute in a microwave on high or finish by quickly searing on each side in a hot oiled skillet.

Roast Pork Stir Fry

NUMBER OF SERVINGS: 4

NUTRITIONAL VALUES PER SERVING: 12.6 grams of carb, 20.1 grams of protein

2	tablespoons coconut or peanut oil
2	cups roasted pork, cut into 1-inch cubes
2	onions, cut into chunks
2	tablespoons soy sauce
1	ounce unsweetened pineapple juice
¾	pound fresh asparagus, cut into 1-inch lengths
⅓	cup fresh mushrooms, sliced
½	cup tomato, chopped
1	teaspoon cornstarch
¼	cup white wine or vinegar

Heat oil in a wok or skillet.

Combine pork, onions, and soy sauce in skillet.

Cook on high heat for 1 or 2 minutes.

Add pineapple juice, asparagus, and mushrooms.

Cook for 5 or 6 minutes more.

Add tomato.

Dissolve cornstarch in white wine or vinegar, and blend into meat mixture, stirring constantly for 2 or 3 minutes until sauce thickens and vegetables are tender.

Hobo Dinner Pork Chops

NUMBER OF SERVINGS: 4

NUTRITIONAL VALUES PER SERVING: 17.5 grams of carb, 48.0 grams of protein

4	pork chops
2	carrots
2	small zucchini squash
1	onion
½	head cauliflower
8	tablespoons concentrate cream of celery soup

Cut 4 12-inch squares of aluminum foil.

Spray foil squares lightly with no-stick cooking spray or grease lightly with coconut oil.

Clean carrots, zucchini squash, onion, and cauliflower and cut into pieces.

Season pork chops to taste, and place one in the center of each foil square.

Top each pork chop with 2 tablespoons of cream of celery soup concentrate and ¼ of each kind of fresh vegetable.

Bring corners of foil up to center and seal seams to make "tents."

Store in refrigerator until cooking time.

Place tents on cookie sheet and bake at 400° for 45 to 50 minutes.

Stuffed Veal

NUMBER OF SERVINGS: 4

NUTRITIONAL VALUES PER SERVING: 2.6 grams of carb, 42.8 grams of protein

- 4   veal cutlets
- ½   teaspoon salt (approximately)
- 4   slices boiled ham
- 6   slices Swiss cheese
- 1   egg, well-beaten
- ¼   cup Parmesan cheese, grated
- 4   tablespoons butter
- ¼   cup dry white wine
     (you'll also need some string)

Preheat oven to 350°.

Wash veal cutlets and pound flat.

Season with salt and pepper to taste.

Top cutlets with boiled ham (one slice each) and Swiss cheese (one slice each).

Roll up and tie with string.

Dip rolls in well-beaten egg.

Roll in Parmesan cheese.

Melt butter in a skillet.

Sauté veal rolls until brown all around.

Place in an oven-proof dish.

Pour on remaining liquid from pan.

Add white wine.

Top with 2 slices of Swiss cheese.

Bake at 350° for 30 minutes.

Remove strings and serve.

Venison Tenderloin with Creamy Rosemary Sauce

NUMBER OF SERVINGS: 4

NUTRITIONAL VALUES PER SERVING: 1.2 grams of carb, 40 grams of protein

2	¾-pound venison tenderloins* (up to 1 pound works)
½	teaspoon salt
½	teaspoon black pepper
½	teaspoon dried parsley flakes
2	teaspoons dried rosemary, crushed (divided use)
1½	cups water
½	cup half-and-half

Preheat the oven to 350°. Lightly grease a roasting pan with coconut oil. Rinse the meat under cool tap water and pat dry. Rub the tenderloins with the salt and pepper and dust with the parsley flakes and 1 teaspoon of the rosemary. Place the tenderloins into the roasting pan, add ½ cup of water to the pan to prevent sticking, and roast uncovered at 350° for 45 minutes. At about 20 minutes, add another ½ cup of water to the roasting pan and continue roasting.

Check for doneness with a meat thermometer: 130° for rare and 140° for medium rare. If necessary continue roasting for another 5 or 6 minutes and check again. Do not overcook game meat or it will become tough. Remove tenderloins from pan and set aside, covered in aluminum foil to keep warm. Pour the pan drippings into a saucepan, scraping up all the brown bits that cling to the pan for added flavor. Add the other ½ cup water and bring to a boil. Reduce heat to low, add the remaining 1 teaspoon of rosemary, and continue to simmer for about ten minutes. Stir in the cream and heat through. Cut into half-inch medallions; top with sauce.

---

*Venison tenderloins are available nationwide from New West Foods or on the Internet at www.NewWestFoods.com. Our thanks to New West Foods for this recipe.

Roasted Paprika Chicken

NUMBER OF SERVINGS: 4

NUTRITIONAL VALUES PER SERVING: 0.9 gram of carb, 39.0 grams of protein

1   whole roasting hen
1 to 2 tablespoons olive oil
2   teaspoons salt
2   teaspoons pepper
1   whole onion
    paprika

Spray roasting pan with no stick cooking spray or grease lightly with coconut oil.

Wash and drain roasting hen.

Brush olive oil onto roasting hen.

Rub salt and pepper onto roasting hen and into cavity.

Peel and quarter onion; place into cavity.

Sprinkle roasting hen liberally with paprika.

Place in roasting pan.

Cover with foil and bake 400° for 45 minutes.

Uncover and bake another 15 minutes or until skin is crisp.

Sunday Spicy Chicken

NUMBER OF SERVINGS: 8

NUTRITIONAL VALUES PER SERVING: 1.6 grams of carb, 58.7 grams of protein

- 4 pounds chicken, cut in pieces
  olive oil, for brushing
- ½ cup light (low-carb) bread crumbs
- ¼ teaspoon thyme
- ½ teaspoon paprika
- ¼ teaspoon salt
- ¼ teaspoon marjoram
- ¼ teaspoon celery seed
- ¼ teaspoon black pepper

Preheat oven to 375°.

Brush chicken pieces with olive oil.

In a large bowl, combine bread crumbs, thyme, paprika, salt, marjoram, celery seed, and black pepper.

Dredge chicken pieces in the coating.

Arrange them on a nonstick baking sheet.

Bake at 375° for 45 minutes until crisp on outside.

Cinder's Lemon Chicken

NUMBER OF SERVINGS: 4 to 6

NUTRITIONAL VALUES PER SERVING: 3.0 grams of carb, 59.3 grams of protein

3	pounds chicken pieces
	salt and pepper, to taste
2	large lemons, cut into wedges
1	onion, cut into chunks
1	garlic clove, minced
1	teaspoon thyme
1	teaspoon marjoram
1	teaspoon pepper
1	tablespoon fresh parsley, chopped
⅓	cup olive oil

Wash chicken pieces.

Arrange chicken pieces in a baking dish.

Sprinkle with salt, pepper, and the juice from the lemons.

Lay juiced lemon wedges on top of chicken pieces.

In a separate bowl, combine onion, garlic, thyme, marjoram, pepper, parsley, and olive oil.

Pour this mixture over the chicken pieces.

Cover and marinate in the refrigerator for several hours.

Allow chicken to come to room temperature and preheat oven to 350°.

Bake, uncovered, for 1½ hours.

Tabasco Chicken

NUMBER OF SERVINGS: 6

NUTRITIONAL VALUES PER SERVING: 0.2 gram of carb, 39.0 grams of protein

1	3-pound chicken, cut up
1	teaspoon Krazy Mixed-up Salt or seasoned salt
¼	teaspoon Tabasco sauce
½	teaspoon paprika
2	tablespoons lime juice
2	tablespoons olive oil

Preheat oven to 350°.

Wash and dry chicken.

Combine Krazy Mixed-up Salt, Tabasco sauce, paprika, lime juice, and olive oil.

Place chicken in a baking dish.

Pour Tabasco mixture over chicken.

Marinate in refrigerator at least 2 hours.

Bring to room temperature before cooking.

Bake at 350° for 1 hour, turning once and basting every 10 minutes.

Barbecued Chicken Wings

NUMBER OF SERVINGS: 10 to 12

NUTRITIONAL VALUES PER SERVING: 1.4 grams of carb, 38.2 grams of protein

- 1   cup water
- ½   cup olive oil
- ½   cup vinegar
- 2   tablespoons chili powder
- ½   cup cayenne pepper
- 5 to 6 pounds chicken wings
-      salt and pepper, to taste

Make a dipping sauce as follows:

In a saucepan, mix together water, olive oil, vinegar, chili powder, and cayenne pepper

Bring to a boil.

Continue boiling 5 minutes, then set aside.

Chop tips from chicken wings.

Sprinkle lightly with salt and pepper.

Cover.

Bring coals of a covered grill to medium-hot heat.

Arrange wings on grill. Cover and smoke.

Turn wings and rearrange frequently to prevent burning.

Cook until wings seem a bit dry (about 1 to 1½ hours).

Remove wings from grill with tongs and immediately dip them into dipping sauce and place onto serving platter.

Rosemary Chicken

NUMBER OF SERVINGS: 4

NUTRITIONAL VALUES PER SERVING: 0.8 gram of carb, 58.5 grams of protein

- 4 medium-sized chicken breast halves, (about 2 pounds)
- 1 tablespoon extra-virgin olive oil
- 2 tablespoons red wine vinegar
- ¼ teaspoon dried rosemary
- ¼ teaspoon dried thyme
- ¼ teaspoon dried tarragon
  dash paprika
  dash black pepper

Coat boiler pan with no-stick cooking spray or grease lightly with coconut oil.

Wash chicken breasts and pat dry. Season lightly with salt.

In a bowl, mix oil, vinegar, rosemary, thyme, tarragon, paprika, and black pepper.

Place chicken breasts in the broiler pan, bone-side down, and brush with marinade.

Broil 6 inches from the heat for 20 minutes.

Turn breasts over and brush with the marinade.

Broil 10 more minutes.

Brush with marinade again.

Broil 5 more minutes.

Grilled Chicken Breasts with Mustard

NUMBER OF SERVINGS: 4

NUTRITIONAL VALUES PER SERVING: 1.7 grams of carb, 30.4 grams of protein

      4   chicken breast halves, skin on
      ¼   cup Dijon mustard
      ¼   cup old-style mustard with seeds
      ¼   cup hot German mustard
      ¼   cup white wine vinegar
      ¼   cup extra-virgin olive oil
      4   packets Splenda
           lemon juice from ½ lemon
      1   shallot, sliced (or substitute ½ onion)
           black pepper, coarsely ground, to taste

Wash chicken breasts and pat dry.

In a separate bowl, mix the three types of mustard, vinegar, olive oil, sweetener, lemon juice, and shallot.

Add pepper to taste.

Marinate chicken breasts at least 3 hours in the refrigerator before grilling.

Grill over medium-hot to red-hot coals for 6 to 7 minutes per side.

Warm the remaining marinade to serve as sauce over chicken.

Skillet Chicken Italiano

NUMBER OF SERVINGS: 4

NUTRITIONAL VALUES PER SERVING: 6.6 grams of carb, 31.6 grams of protein

> 3 tablespoons coconut oil
> 1 clove garlic, minced
> 2 large chicken breasts, skinned and boned, cut into 1-inch cubes
> 1 cup frozen Italian green beans, thawed
> ½ red bell pepper, chopped
> ½ teaspoon salt
> 2 whole tomatoes, quartered
> 4 mashed anchovies, (made to paste)
> 2 tablespoons pimiento, diced
> 1 tablespoon capers, rinsed, drained
> 1 to 2 tablespoons fresh lemon juice

Heat coconut oil in a wok or large skillet over high heat.

Sauté garlic in the oil.

Add chicken breasts, green beans, red pepper, and salt.

Stir-fry for about 3 minutes.

Add tomatoes, anchovies, pimiento, and capers.

Stir-fry for about 1 minute.

Sprinkle with lemon juice.

Turn onto platter and serve.

Roman-Style Chicken

NUMBER OF SERVINGS: 6

NUTRITIONAL VALUES PER SERVING: 8.0 grams of carb, 30.0 grams of protein

6	large chicken breasts *or* thighs
1	onion
4	tablespoons butter
4	tablespoons olive oil
1	14½-ounce can tomatoes, chopped, with the juice
½	teaspoon garlic powder
1	tablespoon sweet basil
½	teaspoon oregano
1	bell pepper
½	pound fresh mushrooms
4	medium zucchini squash
¼	cup Parmesan cheese, grated

Wash and pat dry. Season chicken breasts *or* thighs lightly with salt and pepper. Set aside.

Chop onion, and sauté in 2 tablespoons butter and 2 tablespoons olive oil.

Add chicken breasts and continue cooking until chicken browns slightly.

Add canned tomatoes and juice, garlic powder, basil, and oregano.

Cover and simmer for 20 minutes.

Meanwhile, clean and cut bell pepper into medium strips.

Wash and slice mushrooms and zucchini squash.

In a second pan, sauté bell pepper, 2 tablespoons butter and 2 tablespoons olive oil until pepper is soft.

Add mushrooms and zucchini. Sauté until mushrooms shrink and absorb butter and oil.

Add this mixture to the chicken.

Cover again and simmer another 20 minutes.

Remove from heat.

Stir in grated Parmesan cheese.

Chicken Divan

NUMBER OF SERVINGS: 6

NUTRITIONAL VALUES PER SERVING: 4.8 grams of carb, 18.1 grams of protein

- 1¼ pounds broccoli
- 12 ounces chicken breast, cooked
- ¼ Crème Fraîche*
- ⅛ teaspoon nutmeg
- ⅛ teaspoon pepper
- 1½ teaspoon instant chicken bouillon granules
- ¼ cup Parmesan cheese, grated
  paprika to garnish

Preheat oven to 350°.

Steam broccoli florets until crisp/tender.

Drain and reserve cooking liquid.

Spray an 8-inch baking with no-stick spray or grease lightly with coconut oil.

Arrange broccoli in baking dish.

Slice chicken breast thinly and set aside.

In a saucepan, heat reserved cooking liquid plus water if needed to make 1 cup.

Stir in crème fraîche, nutmeg, pepper, and chicken bouillon granules.

Stir until thickened.

Pour half the sauce over the broccoli.

Layer sliced chicken on top.

Pour remaining sauce over chicken.

Sprinkle with Parmesan cheese.

Use paprika to garnish.

Bake covered at 350° until bubbly, about 25 minutes.

Tuna or Chicken Salad

NUMBER OF SERVINGS: 2

NUTRITIONAL VALUES PER SERVING: 1.9 grams of carb, 33.7 grams of protein

2	eggs
1	6-ounce can tuna or chicken, drained well
5	dill pickle slices, chopped
½	teaspoon garlic powder
2	teaspoons onion, dried, minced (rehydrated)
1½	tablespoons Homemade Mayonnaise*, or to taste
1	tablespoon Dijon-style mustard, or to taste
	sliced tomato (optional)

Hard-boil the eggs, cool, peel, chop, and put into a mixing bowl.

Add to bowl tuna or chicken, eggs, pickle, garlic powder, onion, mayonnaise and mustard.

Variation: Stuffed Tomato   Remove stem from a medium tomato, turn it upside down and slice in wedges from the bottom almost through. Fan the attached wedges into a "star." Fill the center with tuna, chicken, shrimp, or crab salad. (Adds about 4 grams of carb.)

Halibut Jardinière

NUMBER OF SERVINGS: 8

NUTRITIONAL VALUES PER SERVING: 2.9 grams of carb, 20.7 grams of protein

⅔	cup onion, thinly sliced
8	halibut steaks
⅓	cup tomato, chopped
⅓	cup green pepper, chopped
¼	cup fresh parsley, chopped
3	tablespoons pimiento, chopped
1½	cups fresh mushrooms, chopped
⅓	cup dry white wine
2	tablespoons lime juice
1	teaspoon salt
¼	teaspoon dillweed
¼	teaspoon black pepper
	lime, wedges or slices

Preheat oven to 350°.

Spray a baking dish with no-stick cooking spray or grease lightly with coconut oil.

Line bottom of dish with onion slices.

Place halibut steaks on top of onion slices.

In a separate bowl, combine tomato, green pepper, parsley, pimiento, and mushrooms.

Spread mixture over fish steaks.

In a separate bowl, blend wine, lime juice, salt, dillweed, and black pepper.

Pour over fish and vegetables.

Bake at 350° for 25 minutes until fish flakes with a fork.

Garnish with lime wedges or slices.

Fish and Peppers

NUMBER OF SERVINGS: 4

NUTRITIONAL VALUES PER SERVING: 1.7 grams of carb, 15.5 grams of protein

- 1   pound sole *or* flounder fillets
- 1   canned green chili pepper, seeded and minced
- 2   cloves garlic, minced
- 2   tablespoons lemon juice
- 3   tablespoons butter, softened
- 1   tablespoon parsley, minced
- ½   teaspoon black pepper

Preheat broiler.

Wash fillets and pat dry.

Mix green chili pepper, garlic, lemon juice, butter, parsley, and black pepper. Blend well.

Spread pepper mixture evenly on both sides of fillets.

Marinate for 20 minutes.

Broil for 10 minutes or until flaky.

Grilled Salmon Steaks with Chive Butter

NUMBER OF SERVINGS: 4

NUTRITIONAL VALUES PER SERVING: 0.6 gram of carb, 27.2 grams of protein

> 4   1-inch thick (6-ounce) salmon steaks
>   olive oil
> 8   tablespoons (1 stick) butter
>   dash lemon juice
> 1   teaspoon fresh parsley, minced
> 1   tablespoon fresh chives, minced
>   salt and pepper to taste

Salmon

Brush salmon with olive oil.

Grill over medium-hot coals on an open grill about 5 to 6 minutes per side.

Place a pat of chive butter onto each hot steak to serve.

Chive Butter

Allow stick of butter to soften in a bowl until malleable.

With a fork, blend in: a dash of lemon juice, parsley, chives, and salt and pepper to taste.

Form the butter into a 6-inch-long log on a sheet of waxed paper.

Wrap securely and refrigerate until hardened. Use as needed.

Makes about 12 to 15 pats of butter.

Salmon in Tomato Tubs

NUMBER OF SERVINGS: 6

NUTRITIONAL VALUES PER SERVING: 4.3 grams of carb, 19.5 grams of protein

1	13-ounce can pink salmon, drained, all bones and skin removed
2	tablespoons green bell pepper, finely chopped
2	tablespoons green onions, minced green and white parts
2	eggs, beaten
¾	cup half-and-half
2	tablespoons lemon juice (about 1 small lemon)
½	teaspoon salt
¼	teaspoon red pepper flakes
½	teaspoon Worcestershire sauce
6	medium tomatoes
2	tablespoons Parmesan cheese, grated

In a small bowl, wilt onions and peppers, covered with waxed paper, in the microwave on high for 2 minutes. Place the fish into a separate mixing bowl and flake with a fork. Add the onions, peppers, chopped eggs, half and half, lemon juice, salt, red pepper flakes, and Worcestershire sauce and stir to combine with the salmon. Turn the salmon mixture out onto a microwave-safe pie plate or baking dish. Cover loosely with waxed paper and microwave on high for 5 minutes, stirring occasionally. Cook in additional 1-minute bursts until egg has almost completely cooked (about 2 or 3 minutes more).

Slice the stem end off each tomato and scoop out the pulp with a paring knife and a spoon. Divide the salmon mixture evenly between the 6 tomato tubs, filling the cavity and mounding the salmon up slightly. Sprinkle each filled tub with the grated Parmesan cheese. Place the filled tomato tubs in a glass baking dish, cover lightly with a paper towel, and microwave on high for 2 to 3 minutes.

Charlie's Grilled Whole Fish

NUMBER OF SERVINGS: 6

NUTRITIONAL VALUES PER SERVING: 0.9 gram of carb, 59.3 grams of protein

  2 to 2½-pounds whole fish (trout or red snapper are good), cleaned
  1   lemon, sliced thin
  1   small yellow onion, sliced thin
  4   tablespoons butter
      salt and pepper

Place the cleaned fish on two lengths of heavy aluminum foil about 8 inches longer than the fish. Salt and pepper the cavity. Place a layer of lemon slices, closely packed, down the length of the cavity, top that layer with a similar layer of onion slices. Dot these layers with chunks of butter. Scatter any remaining lemon and onion slices over the top of the fish and dot with butter along the side of the fish. Seal the foil securely around the fish, folding in both ends to make a stable packet. Place on a hot grill and cook for 10 to 15 minutes, flip the packet and cook another 10 to 15 minutes. When done, the skin should pull easily away and the flesh should flake with a fork. Separate the fillets from the bone, divide them in three pieces each, and serve.

Skillet Shrimp

NUMBER OF SERVINGS: 6

NUTRITIONAL VALUES PER SERVING: 4.8 grams of carb, 46.1 grams of protein

   3   pounds medium shrimp, raw, cleaned and peeled
   2   sticks butter
12 ounces Italian Dressing*
   1   lemon, juice only
   1   lime, juice only

Melt butter in a large heavy skillet—do not allow to brown. Add salad dressing and lemon and lime juices. Add shrimp and sauté about 10 minutes, stirring and turning occasionally, until all shrimp are cooked through and opaque. Serve immediately.

Shrimp K-Bobs

NUMBER OF SERVINGS: 4 or 5

NUTRITIONAL VALUES PER SERVING: 12.1 grams of carb, 26.3 grams of protein

- 16   large shrimp, cleaned, peeled and deveined
- 4   small bell peppers, cut into approximately 1-inch squares
- 4   small onions, peeled and quartered
- 16   large whole, fresh mushrooms
- olive oil for brushing
- pepper to taste

On 4 or 5 wooden or metal skewers, arrange shrimp, bell pepper, onion, and mushroom in repeating pattern until skewer is full.

Brush all with olive oil.

Sprinkle with pepper.

Grill over medium- to red-hot coals for 4 minutes a side or until done.

Vegetable Dishes

Asparagus Jayme

NUMBER OF SERVINGS: 2 (4 stalks each)

NUTRITIONAL VALUES PER SERVING: 2.6 grams of carb, 1.6 grams of protein

8	stalks fresh asparagus
2	tablespoons extra-virgin olive oil
1	clove garlic, crushed
2	teaspoons white wine vinegar

Bring water to boil in a shallow pan or skillet.

Wash and trim ends from asparagus.

Place asparagus in boiling water until they turn bright green.

Remove promptly and submerge in cold water to stop the cooking process.

Chill.

Mix the olive oil, garlic, and vinegar. (It is best done ahead and left to sit for several hours to allow garlic to flavor the oil and vinegar.)

Before serving, pour the vinegar and oil over the chilled asparagus.

Asparagus Parmesano

NUMBER OF SERVINGS: 4

NUTRITIONAL VALUES PER SERVING: 4.8 grams of carb, 5.7 grams of protein

1	pound fresh asparagus
1	tablespoon butter
1	tablespoon flour
¼	cup chicken broth
¼	cup milk
2	tablespoons cheddar cheese, shredded
3	tablespoons Parmesan cheese, grated
¼	teaspoon salt
¼	teaspoon pepper

Wash and trim ends from asparagus.

In a skillet, bring water to a boil—enough to cover asparagus.

Cook asparagus in boiling water until just bright green and crisp. Drain, put in serving dish, and keep hot.

In a saucepan, melt butter.

Stir in flour.

Add chicken broth and milk, gradually.

Cook, stirring, until mixture thickens.

Stir in cheddar cheese, 2 of the 3 tablespoons of Parmesan cheese, salt, and pepper.

Pour cheese sauce over asparagus.

Sprinkle with last tablespoon of Parmesan cheese.

Sautéed Broccoli

NUMBER OF SERVINGS: 4

NUTRITIONAL VALUES PER SERVING: 4.1 grams of carb, 2.5 grams of protein

4	teaspoons olive oil
2	garlic cloves, chopped
1	10-ounce package frozen broccoli, thawed
½	cup chicken broth
1	tablespoon fresh lemon juice
¼	teaspoon lemon peel, grated
¼	teaspoon pepper

In a large skillet, heat olive oil.

Sauté garlic.

Add broccoli.

Cook about one minute, stirring occasionally.

Add chicken broth, lemon juice, lemon peel, and pepper.

Reduce heat. Cover and simmer for 5 to 7 minutes until broccoli is crisp-tender.

Matilda's Marinated Green Beans

NUMBER OF SERVINGS: 4 to 6

NUTRITIONAL VALUES PER SERVING: 3.9 grams of carb, 0.8 gram of protein

1	large can French-cut green beans
1	can water chestnuts, chopped
1	can chow mein vegetables
1	can mushrooms, sliced
1	jar pimiento, chopped
$\frac{1}{3}$	cup extra-virgin olive oil
$\frac{1}{4}$	cup wine vinegar
6	packets Splenda
1	teaspoon salt
1	teaspoon pepper
1	teaspoon garlic powder

In a mixing bowl, combine green beans, water chestnuts, chow mein vegetables, mushrooms, and pimiento.

In a separate bowl, stir together olive oil, wine vinegar, sweetener, salt, pepper, and garlic powder.

Pour marinade over vegetables and stir to coat well.

Cover and refrigerate for at least one hour to allow flavors to combine.

Serve cold.

Fancy Green Beans

NUMBER OF SERVINGS: 4 to 6

NUTRITIONAL VALUES PER SERVING: 4.6 grams of carb, 0.9 gram of protein

1   pound fresh green beans
2   tablespoons butter
1   small can water chestnuts, sliced
      salt and pepper, to taste

Wash and trim ends from green beans.

Steam beans 7 to 8 minutes (until they turn bright green).

In a skillet, melt butter.

Add and sauté steamed beans and water chestnuts.

Season with salt and pepper to taste.

Sour Cream Beans

NUMBER OF SERVINGS: 8

NUTRITIONAL VALUES PER SERVING: 4.3 grams of carb, 3.4 grams of protein

2   10-ounce packages frozen French-cut green beans
6   slices bacon, cooked and drained
2   tablespoons bacon drippings
¾   cup sour cream

Cook beans according to package directions. Drain and place beans into medium saucepan. Fry the bacon until crisp, reserving 2 tablespoons of the bacon drippings. In a small mixing bowl, stir bacon drippings into the sour cream and combine well. Add the sour cream to the beans; crumble the bacon into the bean mixture and stir to combine all ingredients. Reheat beans over low heat, stirring occasionally to prevent sticking, until thoroughly hot. Serve immediately.

Sassy Green Beans

NUMBER OF SERVINGS: 3 or 4

NUTRITIONAL VALUES PER SERVING: 5.7 grams of carb, 2.4 grams of protein

¾   pound whole, fresh green beans
3   ounces tomato juice
3   ounces water
2   tablespoons onion, chopped
1   teaspoon oregano
½   teaspoon basil
½   teaspoon garlic powder
¼   teaspoon salt
¼   teaspoon pepper
1   tablespoon Romano cheese, grated

Wash and cut green beans into 1-inch pieces.

In a saucepan, combine the beans, tomato juice, water, onion, oregano, basil, garlic powder, salt, and pepper.

Cover, reduce heat, and simmer for 5 minutes.

Uncover and cook until green beans are tender.

Sprinkle with Romano cheese.

Grilled Zucchini

NUMBER OF SERVINGS: 4 to 6

NUTRITIONAL VALUES PER SERVING: 4.6 grams of carb, 2.0 grams of protein

    4   large zucchini
        olive oil, to brush on zucchini
        salt, a dash
        garlic powder, a dash
        Parmesan cheese, a dash

Clean and trim ends from zucchini, and slice approximately ¼-inch thick, lengthwise.

Brush both sides of cut zucchini with olive oil.

Sprinkle on salt, pepper, garlic powder, and Parmesan cheese.

Grill over medium-hot coals for 10 minutes, turning frequently.

Or broil under oven broiler for 4 to 5 minutes per side.

Italian Zucchini Bake

NUMBER OF SERVINGS: 6

NUTRITIONAL VALUES PER SERVING: 7.0 grams of carb, 3.4 grams of protein

4	large zucchini
2	tablespoons butter
1	clove garlic, minced
1	onion, chopped
2	small tomatoes
2	tablespoons fresh parsley, snipped
⅜	cup cheddar cheese, shredded
	black pepper, to taste

Wash and cut zucchini into rounds.

In a skillet, melt butter.

Add garlic and onion.

Sauté until transparent.

Add the zucchini and sauté about 5 minutes, until tender.

Peel and chop tomatoes.

Add parsley to the tomatoes.

Spray a baking dish with no-stick cooking spray or grease lightly with coconut oil.

Layer tomatoes, then zucchini, then cheddar cheese.

Repeat the layers and sprinkle top with black pepper.

Bake at 350° for 40 minutes.

Zucchini Medley

NUMBER OF SERVINGS: 5 to 6

NUTRITIONAL VALUES PER SERVING: 4.0 grams of carb, 2.1 grams of protein

2	tablespoons butter
1	teaspoon garlic, minced
1	large fresh tomato, diced
1	teaspoon fresh parsley, chopped fine
½	teaspoon oregano
½	teaspoon black pepper, coarsely ground
½	cup water
2	large zucchini, sliced in rounds
1½	cups cauliflower (broken into florets)
2	tablespoons Parmesan *or* Romano cheese

In a large skillet, melt butter.

Sauté garlic until transparent.

Add tomato, parsley, oregano, black pepper, and water.

Cook over medium-high heat for 3 minutes.

Meanwhile, steam zucchini and cauliflower until cooked but still crisp.

Add vegetables to skillet and cook, 5 minutes more, stirring occasionally.

Sprinkle on Parmesan *or* Romano cheese.

Skillet Ratatouille

NUMBER OF SERVINGS: 4

NUTRITIONAL VALUES PER SERVING: 15.4 grams of carb, 3.2 grams of protein

1	large eggplant
4	medium zucchini
1	large white onion
3	cloves garlic
1	large bell pepper
2	large tomatoes
2	tablespoons parsley, chopped
2	tablespoons olive oil
1	teaspoon dried oregano
1	teaspoon dried basil
	salt and pepper, to taste

Clean, peel and coarsely chop the eggplant, zucchini, onion, garlic, bell pepper, tomatoes, and parsley.

In a skillet, heat olive oil.

Sauté onion and garlic until they are transparent.

Add eggplant, zucchini, bell pepper, tomatoes, and parsley.

Season with oregano, basil, and salt and pepper to taste.

Continue to sauté until the vegetables are tender, stirring to prevent sticking.

Eggplant Milano

NUMBER OF SERVINGS: 6

NUTRITIONAL VALUES PER SERVING: 6.4 grams of carb, 1.0 gram of protein

2	tablespoons olive oil
1	eggplant, peeled and coarsely chopped
½	cup celery, thickly sliced
1	onion, coarsely chopped
2	cups tomato, coarsely chopped
¼	cup red wine vinegar
1	teaspoon oregano
¼	teaspoon basil
¼	teaspoon salt
¼	teaspoon pepper

In a skillet, heat olive oil.

Add eggplant, celery, and onion.

Cook over medium heat until onion is transparent.

Add tomato, red wine vinegar, oregano, basil, salt, and pepper.

Cover and simmer for 25 minutes.

Bravely Braised Cabbage

NUMBER OF SERVINGS: 8

NUTRITIONAL VALUES PER SERVING: 2.9 grams of carb, 1.9 grams of protein

    4   cups green cabbage, cut in pieces
    2   cups chicken broth
    2   tablespoons butter
    ½   teaspoon salt (or to taste)
    ½   teaspoon pepper (or to taste)

In a large covered pot, simmer cabbage pieces in chicken broth about 20 minutes or until tender. Uncover and continue to simmer until most of the liquid has boiled away. Add butter, salt, and pepper. Toss to coat leaves evenly. Serve immediately.

Note: if you multiply the recipe, the cooking time may be a bit longer. Just cook until tender as directed.

Tangy Cabbage

NUMBER OF SERVINGS: 2

NUTRITIONAL VALUES PER SERVING: 6.3 grams of carb, 1.9 grams of protein

2	cups cabbage
1	tablespoon butter
¼	cup water
½	teaspoon salt
1	tablespoon white vinegar
2	packets Splenda
½	teaspoon Dijon-style mustard
2	tablespoons sour cream
2	tablespoons Homemade Mayonnaise*

Shred cabbage.

In saucepan, melt butter, add cabbage. Stir to coat with butter.

Add water and salt.

Stir and cover to simmer for 10 minutes.

Drain cabbage and set aside.

Mustard sauce:

In a second saucepan, combine vinegar, sweetener, and mustard.

Cover and simmer on very low heat for 1 minute.

In a bowl, combine sour cream and mayonnaise.

Add the mustard sauce to the sour cream and mayonnaise.

Fold this mixture into cabbage. Stir well to coat.

Cukes and Onions

NUMBER OF SERVINGS: 4

NUTRITIONAL VALUES PER SERVING: 5.2 grams of carb, 0.8 grams of protein

2	cucumbers
2	white onions
1	teaspoon salt
2	tablespoons white vinegar
¼	cup water
1	packet Splenda

Peel cucumbers and onions, slice very thin, and place them into a bowl.

Sprinkle with salt, toss and cover.

Set aside for 1 hour.

Drain off liquid.

In a separate bowl, combine vinegar, water, and sweetener.

Pour vinegar mixture over cucumbers and onions and refrigerate for several hours.

Can be prepared up to 24 hours in advance.

Herbed Brussels Sprouts

NUMBER OF SERVINGS: 4

NUTRITIONAL VALUES PER SERVING: 7.4 grams of carb, 2.4 grams of protein

- 1   10-ounce package frozen Brussels sprouts
- 1   small onion, thinly sliced
- 1   tablespoon butter
- 1   clove garlic, minced
- ¼   teaspoon thyme
- ¼   teaspoon oregano
- ¼   teaspoon salt
- ¼   teaspoon pepper

Steam Brussels sprouts and onion slices for about 10 minutes.

In a saucepan, melt butter.

Sauté garlic until brown, but do not burn.

Add the steamed sprouts and onion, thyme, oregano, salt, and pepper.

Cook, stirring occasionally, for 4 to 5 minutes, until vegetables are heated through.

Sautéed Mushrooms

NUMBER OF SERVINGS: 3

NUTRITIONAL VALUES PER SERVING: 2.6 grams of carb, 1.1 grams of protein

8   ounces sliced white mushrooms
1   tablespoon butter
1   tablespoon olive oil
1   clove garlic, minced or pressed
½   cup dry wine (red or white)
    salt and pepper to taste

Heat butter and oil in a large skillet over medium heat.

Add garlic and allow it to become slightly translucent, but do not brown.

Add the mushrooms and stir to coat with the oil, keeping them moving as they cook.

When the mushrooms become somewhat limp, add the wine. Allow the wine to boil, reducing the liquid by about half, stirring occasionally.

Reduce heat to lowest setting allowing the wine to be almost completely absorbed.

Keep warm until serving.

(Use white wine if you're serving the mushrooms with poultry, pork, veal, or fish and red if you're serving them with beef, lamb, or game.)

Stewart's Mushrooms

NUMBER OF SERVINGS: 3
NUTRITIONAL VALUES PER SERVING: 2.3 grams of carb, 2.3 grams of protein

- 8   ounces fresh mushrooms, cleaned
- 1   cup water
- 1   tablespoon butter
- ½   teaspoon salt
- 2   teaspoons Pickapeppa Sauce

Place mushrooms in a steamer basket over about 1 cup of steaming water. Cover and steam about 10 minutes. Place the butter and Pickapeppa Sauce into a serving bowl. Remove mushrooms from the heat, empty them from the steamer into the serving bowl. Sprinkle with salt; toss gently to coat evenly. Serve immediately.

Vegetarian Dishes

Baked Tofu Caesar Salad

NUMBER OF SERVINGS: 1

NUTRITIONAL VALUES PER SERVING: 6.0 grams of carb for 4 ounces, 9.0 grams
   of carb for 6 ounces, 19.0 grams of protein for 4 ounces, 28.0 grams of
   protein for 6 ounces

   2   cups Romaine lettuce
   1 to 2 tablespoons healthy commercial Caesar dressing
   4 to 6 ounces pre-seasoned, pre-baked tofu, sliced
   1   tablespoon sesame seeds

Toss lettuce with dressing.

Place tofu over dressed lettuce.

Sprinkle sesame seeds over the top and serve.

Veggie Pita TLT

NUMBER OF SERVINGS: 1

NUTRITIONAL VALUES PER SERVING: 17.0 grams of carb, 19.0 grams of protein

½   small pita
    large leaf lettuce
    Homemade Mayonnaise*, to taste
    mustard, to taste
4   ounces pre-seasoned tofu, baked and sliced
½   small tomato, sliced
1   cup sprouts
    sesame seeds, a sprinkle

Line pita with lettuce leaf.

Spread on mayo and mustard.

Fill with tofu slices.

Add tomato slices.

Top with sprouts and sesame seeds.

Veggie-Stuffed Avocado (Tofu and Egg Salad)

NUMBER OF SERVINGS: 2 (serving size ½ cup)

NUTRITIONAL VALUES PER SERVING: 4.4 grams of carb, 19.0 grams of protein

- 4   ounces tofu, pre-cooked
- 2   eggs, hard-boiled
- 2   egg whites, hard-boiled
- 2   tablespoons Homemade Mayonnaise*
- 1   tablespoon spicy mustard
- 1   tablespoon dill pickle relish
- 1   teaspoon onion powder
       salt and pepper, to taste

Dice tofu and eggs and place in medium-sized bowl.

Mix in mayo, mustard, relish, onion powder, salt, and pepper.

Stuff ½ mixture into each avocado half and serve.

Broiled Rosemary Veggie Burger

NUMBER OF SERVINGS: 1

NUTRITIONAL VALUES PER SERVING: The carbohydrates and proteins depend on
brand. Check label.

1 to 2 veggie burger patties, thawed
1   tablespoon butter, softened
½   teaspoon fresh or ¼ teaspoon dried rosemary

Place burgers on the grill, 5 minutes first side and flip, then 4 to 5
minutes more.

Mix butter and rosemary.

Top each burger with herbed butter and continue grilling for
another 5 minutes.

Veggie Tofu Chili

NUMBER OF SERVINGS: 4

NUTRITIONAL VALUES PER SERVING: The carbohydrates and proteins depend on
   veggie protein burger brand. Check label.

   ¼ cup onion, chopped
   ¼ cup bell pepper, diced
   ¼ cup mushrooms, sliced or chopped
       texturized vegetable protein hamburger substitute, equal to
          1 pound ground beef
   1   small can tomatoes, sliced or whole (if whole, cut into pieces)
   2   tablespoons chili powder (or to taste)
       salt

Spray a skillet with no-stick cooking spray or grease lightly with
coconut oil.

Quickly sauté onion and bell pepper, then add and sauté mushrooms. Set aside.

Crumble and brown veggie protein burger and drain fat.

In a deep saucepan or stockpot, combine browned veggie protein
burger, onion, mushrooms, pepper, tomatoes, and enough water to
achieve desired thickness.

Blend in chili powder and salt to taste.

Simmer about 30 minutes.

Cabbage Lasagna

This recipe uses cabbage leaves as a substitute for noodles. Swiss chard will work equally as well.

NUMBER OF SERVINGS: 8

NUTRITIONAL VALUES PER SERVING: About 9 grams of carb plus the amount in
the veggie burger. Protein varies. Check label.

1	medium to large head cabbage
1	tablespoon olive oil
2	cloves garlic, minced or pressed
1	medium onion, chopped
	texturized vegetable protein hamburger substitute, equal to ¾ pound ground beef
1	6-ounce can tomato paste
1	8-ounce can tomato sauce
1	teaspoon oregano, dried
2	teaspoons salt
1	teaspoon black pepper
1	cup mozzarella cheese, grated
½	cup ricotta or cottage cheese
½	cup Parmesan cheese, freshly grated

Preheat the oven to 350°.

Wash cabbage and remove tough outer leaves.

Cut the head in half.

Carefully peel back leaves, trying to keep them intact; these will serve as the lasagna noodles.

Arrange individual leaves on a steamer basket or tray and steam until nearly tender, about 3 to 5 minutes. (You can also do this in the microwave.)

Set aside.

Heat olive oil in a large skillet over medium-high heat.

Sauté garlic, onion, and green pepper until onion is translucent.

Add veggie protein burger. Brown thoroughly.

Drain accumulated fat and water.

Add tomato paste, tomato sauce, and seasonings to the mixture and combine well.

Coat a 9- by 13- by 2-inch baking pan with a little olive oil or coconut oil.

Line the bottom with a layer of cabbage leaves.

Top with half the veggie protein burger mixture.

Add a third of the mozzarella and half of the ricotta cheese.

Add another layer of cabbage leaves, the remaining half of the veggie protein burger mixture, another third of the mozzarella, and the remaining half of the ricotta.

Top with the remaining mozzarella and finish by scattering the Parmesan on top.

Bake, covered, for about 20 minutes. Uncover and bake for 5 minutes more.

Note: can also be made with ¾ pound ground beef for a non-veggie lasagna.

Tofu and Broccoli Frittata

NUMBER OF SERVINGS: 4

NUTRITIONAL VALUES PER SERVING: 3.0 grams of carb, 15.3 grams of protein

4 to 6 ounces tofu
1   cup broccoli, cooked
½   cup roasted red peppers
⅓   cup feta cheese
4   extra-large eggs
     salt and pepper, to taste
2   tablespoons olive oil or butter
½   cup Parmesan cheese, grated

Mix eggs in a bowl with salt and pepper, using a fork.

Heat oil or butter in a 10-inch ovenproof skillet.

Pour eggs into the skillet.

Scatter broccoli and roasted red peppers over the eggs in the skillet.

Crumble feta cheese on top.

Cook the frittata over medium heat until the bottom sets.

Sprinkle cheese over the top, then run it under the broiler until golden brown.

Desserts and Preserves

Mango Smoothie

NUMBER OF SERVINGS: 1

NUTRITIONAL VALUES PER SERVING: 15.1 grams of carb plus that contributed by protein powder, 8.0 grams of protein plus that contributed by protein powder

½   cup mango, diced
2   tablespoons sour cream
1   cup unsweetened soy milk
     protein powder
½   teaspoon vanilla extract
1   packet Splenda
     lime zest of 1 lime
     dash salt
¾   cup water

Mix together all ingredients in a blender until smooth and drink immediately.

Variation: Substitute your favorite berries or melon for the mango to reduce carb to under 10 grams total.

Orange and Strawberry Cup

NUMBER OF SERVINGS: 3

NUTRITIONAL VALUES PER SERVING: 5.0 grams of carb, 0 grams of protein

1   valencia orange, peeled and sectioned
1   cup fresh or frozen, unsweetened strawberries, sliced

Cut orange sections into 3 or 4 pieces each.

Combine with sliced berries.

Chill and serve (½ cup each).

Strawberry Cheesecake

NUMBER OF SERVINGS: 6 to 8

NUTRITIONAL VALUES PER SERVING: 3.4 grams of carb, 4.0 grams of protein

8	ounces cream cheese
4	ounces half-and-half
4	packets Splenda
2	eggs
2	teaspoons vanilla extract
1	cup strawberries, sliced
½	cup sour cream

Preheat oven to 350°.

In a blender or food processor, combine cream cheese, half-and-half, 3 packets of sweetener, eggs and vanilla extract.

Blend until completely smooth.

Pour into an 8-inch ceramic or Pyrex pie pan.[†]

Bake for 25 minutes.

Chill well.

Garnish with sliced strawberries and sour cream (to which 1 packet sweetener is added).

[†]Use a Simple Nut Crust* if desired for an additional 3.8 grams per serving.

Mini Chocolate Chip Cheesecakes

NUMBER OF SERVINGS: 12

NUTRITIONAL VALUES PER SERVING: 2.2 grams of carb, 2.4 grams of protein

- 8 tablespoons finely chopped pecans
- 2 packets Splenda
- 1 tablespoon butter, melted
- 1 large egg, beaten
- 8 ounces cream cheese, softened
- ¼ cup Splenda (granular)
- ¼ teaspoon vanilla extract
- 2 tablespoons semi-sweet mini chocolate chips

Place the nuts, the 2 packets of Splenda, and the butter in a small bowl and combine thoroughly. Line the 12 wells of a muffin tin with paper cupcake liners and distribute the nut mixture evenly among them (about 2 teaspoons per well).

Place the egg, granular Splenda, cream cheese, and vanilla extract into a blender or food processor and blend until smooth. Fold in the chocolate chips. Divide the mixture evenly among the 12 cups. Bake for 15 minutes at 350°. Cool and refrigerate at least one hour. Will keep refrigerated for several days.

Simple Nut Crust for Desserts

NUMBER OF SERVINGS: 8 (one 8-inch crust)

NUTRITIONAL VALUES PER SERVING: 3.8 grams of carb, 1.4 grams of protein

1¼ cups pecans *or* walnuts, ground
4   packets Splenda
2   tablespoons flour
⅛   tablespoon salt
2   tablespoons melted butter

Preheat oven to 375°.

In a bowl, combine all ingredients.

Chill for 30 minutes.

Press mixture into an 8-inch pie plate.

Bake for 10 minutes.

Cool and fill.

Chocolate Butter Wafers

NUMBER OF SERVINGS: about 20 (1 piece each)

NUTRITIONAL VALUES PER SERVING: 1.0 gram of carb, 0.6 gram of protein

8	tablespoons (1 stick) butter
⅓	cup cocoa
½	cup instant nonfat dry milk powder
1	ounce Gulf Wax canning paraffin
1	teaspoon vanilla
14	packets Splenda

In a mixing bowl, soften butter.

Add cocoa and instant nonfat dry milk powder and mix well.

Lay out a 36-inch piece of waxed paper on counter.

In the top of a double boiler, melt canning paraffin.

Add butter, milk, and cocoa mixture.

Begin to whisk constantly with a wire whisk as mixture dissolves.

When totally blended, remove from heat.

Add vanilla and sweetener.

Drop by spoonfuls onto waxed paper.

Stir mixture a bit after each spoonful.

Allow to cool for 30 minutes.

Place on platter lined with waxed paper, separating layers with more waxed paper.

Refrigerate.

Meringue Tart Shells

NUMBER OF SERVINGS: 6

NUTRITIONAL VALUES PER SERVING: 3.1 grams of carb (unfilled), 3.8 grams of
protein

3	egg whites
¼	teaspoon salt
3	packets Splenda
1	teaspoon vanilla extract
½	cup almond meal
¼	cup almonds, coarsely ground
	Filling: any no-bake, sugar-free, aspartame-free filling or fruit and cream.

Preheat oven to 250°.

In a bowl, combine egg whites, salt, sweetener, and vanilla extract. Beat until stiff.

Fold in almond meal and ground almonds.

Drop by large spoonfuls onto buttered cookie sheet.

Create a depression in each mound with the bottom of a glass.

Bake for 30 minutes, then turn off heat, but leave oven door closed for another 30 minutes.

Fill with any no-bake, sugar-free, aspartame-free filling or fruit and cream.

Hot Chocolate

NUMBER OF SERVINGS: 1

NUTRITIONAL VALUES PER SERVING: 3.3 grams of carb, 1.2 grams of protein

- 1   teaspoon baking cocoa
- 1   packet Splenda
     dash salt *or* NoSalt
     dash cinnamon
- 5   ounces boiling water
- ½ ounce half-and-half
     whipped heavy cream sweetened with Splenda (1 packet)

In a cup or mug, place baking cocoa, sweetener, salt *or* NoSalt, and cinnamon.

Add boiling water and half-and-half. Stir well.

Top with sweetened whipped cream.

Strawberry Preserves

NUMBER OF SERVINGS: about 64 (1 tablespoon each)

NUTRITIONAL VALUES PER SERVING: 0.9 gram of carb, 0.1 gram of protein

    1   quart fresh strawberries
    1   lemon
    2   envelopes unflavored gelatin
    ½   cup water
    10   packets Splenda

Rinse, stem, and quarter strawberries.

Place them into saucepan and add the juice of 1 lemon.

Cover and simmer until berries soften and give up their juice.

Meanwhile, in a separate bowl, dissolve unflavored gelatin for 1 minute in ½ cup water.

Add gelatin mixture to berries and remove from heat.

With electric mixer on low speed, mix in sweetener.

Pour into storage jar or container.

Refrigerate uncovered for 2 hours, then stir well, and cover.

Refrigerate again for at least 12 hours to set.

Use as needed.

Store in refrigerator. Will keep for several weeks.

Mixed-Berry Syrup

NUMBER OF SERVINGS: 4

NUTRITIONAL VALUES PER SERVING: 2.6 grams of carb, 0.2 gram of protein

1   cup frozen mixed berries, unsweetened (thawed)
½   cup water
½   teaspoon guar gum[†]
4   packets Splenda or Stevia

Puree thawed berries, water, and sweetener in the blender. Pour into a small saucepan, stir in the guar gum, and warm the mixture over medium-low heat until it thickens. Add a bit of water if too thick or a tiny bit more guar gum if too thin. Serve warm.

You can substitute all raspberries, all strawberries, and all black-berries for a slightly lower-carb cost per serving. Substituting all blue-berries will increase the carb-per-serving only slightly.

[†]Guar gum is a fiber thickener that will not increase the effective carb count of your recipes. Available at www.vitamincottage.com.

Condiments

Red Wine Vinaigrette

NUMBER OF SERVINGS: 6 (10-ounce servings)

NUTRITIONAL VALUES PER SERVING: >1.0 gram of carb, 0 grams of protein

   ¼   cup red wine vinegar
   If herbs are dry, use half as much.
   ½   teaspoon fresh basil
   ½   teaspoon fresh chive
   ½   teaspoon fresh parsley, chopped
   1   small garlic clove
   ½   cup virgin olive oil
   ¼   teaspoon each, salt and pepper, if desired

Pour vinegar into a bowl, whisk in herbs.

Add salt and pepper if desired.

Let stand.

Just before serving, whisk in olive oil in a slow, steady stream.

Roquefort Dressing

NUMBER OF SERVINGS: 7 (1 ounce each)

NUTRITIONAL VALUES PER SERVING: 1.2 grams of carb, 2.3 grams of protein

½ cup sour cream
2 tablespoons wine vinegar
¼ teaspoon tarragon
1 packet Splenda
1 teaspoon Krazy Mixed-Up Salt *or* seasoned salt
½ teaspoon celery seed
2 ounces Roquefort cheese, crumbled, divided use.

In a blender, combine all ingredients except 1 ounce Roquefort cheese.

Blend well until dressing is smooth in consistency.

Carefully fold in rest of crumbled Roquefort cheese.

Store in a container with a tight-fitting lid.

Italian Dressing

NUMBER OF SERVINGS: 8 (1 ounce each)

NUTRITIONAL VALUES PER SERVING: 1.6 grams of carb, 0.1 gram of protein
(Recipe doubles well)

- 1   teaspoon rosemary leaves
- ½   teaspoon salt
- 1   teaspoon garlic powder
- 1   teaspoon ground oregano
- 1   teaspoon basil leaves
- 3   red and 3 black peppercorns
- ¼   teaspoon dill weed (or less if you're not fond of dill)
- ⅓   cup wine vinegar
- ⅔   cup olive oil
- 1   lemon

With a mortar and pestle, pulverize rosemary leaves and salt.

Add and pulverize garlic powder, oregano, basil, peppercorns, and dillweed.

Add spices to wine vinegar.

Let stand for 30 minutes.

Add olive oil and the juice of one lemon.

Mix well and store in cruet or jar.

Flavor is fullest if you do not refrigerate.

Tangy French Dressing

NUMBER OF SERVINGS: 15 (1 ounce each)

NUTRITIONAL VALUES PER SERVING: 0.8 gram of carb, 0.6 gram of protein

3	teaspoons Krazy Mixed-Up Salt *or* seasoned salt
½	teaspoon dry mustard
1	packet Splenda
1	teaspoon Dijon-style mustard
1½	teaspoons lemon juice
1	teaspoon garlic powder
¼	teaspoon tarragon, dried
½	cup olive oil
1	raw egg, well beaten[†]
½	cup heavy cream

In a blender or shaker jar with a tight-fitting lid, combine all ingredients.

Shake until well blended.

Chill 1 hour to blend flavors.

Store in a jar or cruet with a tight-fitting lid.

[†]A note of caution: In recipes calling for raw eggs, the eggs in their shells should be immersed in boiling water for 30 seconds prior to their use.

Minted Yogurt Dressing

NUMBER OF SERVINGS: 6 (about ¾ cup total)

NUTRITIONAL VALUES PER SERVING (about 2 tablespoons): 1.3 grams of carb,
1.0 gram of protein

- ½ cup plain unsweetened yogurt
- 2 tablespoons heavy cream
- ¼ cup water
- 3 tablespoons fresh mint, finely chopped
- ¼ teaspoon garlic powder
- salt and pepper to taste

Blend all ingredients together on low speed. Pour into a tight-sealing container and refrigerate for at least one hour to blend flavors. Will keep in refrigerator for several days.

Homemade Mayonnaise

NUMBER OF SERVINGS: 16 (1 tablespoon each)
NUTRITIONAL VALUES PER SERVING: 0.2 gram of carb, 0.4 gram of protein

1   raw egg[†]
1   teaspoon dry mustard
1   teaspoon salt
    dash cayenne pepper
1   packet Splenda
¼   cup olive oil
¾ to 1 cup light olive oil
3   tablespoons lemon juice

In a blender on high, blend egg, dry mustard, salt, cayenne pepper, sweetener, and ¼ cup olive oil.

With blender running, add in a very slow stream, ½ cup light olive oil, and then lemon juice.

Then, very slowly add an additional ¼ to ½ cup light olive oil.

Stop blender to stir down if necessary.

Store in a jar with a tight-fitting lid.

[†]A note of caution: In recipes calling for raw eggs, the eggs in their shells should be immersed in boiling water for 30 seconds prior to their use.

Crème Fraîche

NUMBER OF SERVINGS: about 1 cup (8 servings)

NUTRITIONAL VALUES PER SERVING: 0.9 gram of carb, 0.6 gram of protein

1 cup heavy cream
1 teaspoon cultured buttermilk

Warm the cream very gently in a small saucepan (over low heat) to just under 100°. Add the buttermilk and stir to combine. Pour the cream into a container with a tight-fitting lid and allow it to sit on the counter near the stove or in a warm place overnight (at least 12 hours) until it thickens. Stir and refrigerate. It will keep for up to 1 week in the refrigerator.

Blender Hollandaise Sauce

NUMBER OF SERVINGS: 4 to 6

NUTRITIONAL VALUES PER SERVING: 0.5 gram of carb, 1.4 grams of protein

    8   tablespoons (1 stick) unsalted butter
    3   egg yolks (reserve whites for another use, if desired)
    2   tablespoons fresh lemon juice
        dash cayenne pepper

In a small saucepan, melt butter.

Meanwhile, in a blender, blend egg yolks, lemon juice, and cayenne pepper.

With blender running, add melted butter in a slow stream.

The sauce should thicken as you blend another 30 or 45 seconds.

Serve immediately.

Dry Rub for Meats

NUMBER OF SERVINGS: makes enough for many barbecues
NUTRITIONAL VALUES PER SERVING: 2.5 grams of carb, 0.1 gram of protein

$\frac{1}{2}$ cup black pepper
$\frac{1}{2}$ cup paprika
$\frac{1}{2}$ cup brown sugar
1   tablespoon garlic powder
1   tablespoon onion powder
1   tablespoon cayenne pepper

In a zip closure bag, combine all ingredients and shake to mix.
Store dry rub in an airtight zip bag or jar.

Use by rubbing a few tablespoons onto meats to season them prior
to barbecuing.

Excellent on ribs, brisket, pork roasts, and chicken.

Versatile Meat Marinade

NUTRITIONAL VALUES PER SERVING: 4.0 grams of carb, 2.1 grams of protein

- ½   cup extra-virgin olive oil
- ⅛   cup red wine vinegar
- 1   teaspoon garlic, minced
- 1   teaspoon black pepper
- 1   teaspoon Cavender's Seasoning

In a zip closure bag or jar, mix all ingredients.

If using for chops, steak, chicken breasts, or thick fish fillets, you may place frozen pieces directly into the zip-closure bag and defrost while marinating in the refrigerator overnight.

If cooking and marinating the same day, you will want to allow at least an hour or so at room temperature to impart flavor to the meat before grilling or baking.

Mr. Ron's Barbecue Sauce

NUMBER OF SERVINGS: 84 (1 ounce each)

NUTRITIONAL VALUES PER SERVING: 2.8 grams of carb, 0.3 gram of protein

42   ounces Dia-Mel or Featherweight Diet Catsup[†] (1 gram of carb per tablespoon)
32   ounces white vinegar
1   10-ounce can tomato puree
1   medium white onion, chopped
6   tablespoons salt
6   tablespoons black pepper
6   tablespoons chili powder
6   tablespoons Splenda

In a large heavy stockpot, combine all ingredients.

Simmer for 4 to 6 hours.

Pour into sterilized canning jars and seal while hot.

[†]Made with Muir Glen Organic regular catsup, carb increases to 4.1 grams per ounce.

Appendix A

Carbohydrate Content of Combination Foods (Dairy, Nuts, Soy)

Milk

Whole	8 ounces	11 grams
2%	8 ounces	12 grams
1%	8 ounces	13 grams
Nonfat	8 ounces	12 grams
Buttermilk	8 ounces	12 grams
Goat's	8 ounces	11 grams
Evaporated milk	2 tablespoons	3 grams

Yogurt

Plain	8 ounces	12 to 17 grams
Flavored	8 ounces	30 to 50 grams

Cream

Half and half	8 ounces	8 grams
	1 tablespoon	0.5 grams
Light	8 ounces	7 grams
	1 tablespoon	0.4 grams
Heavy	8 ounces	6 grams
	1 tablespoon	0.3 grams

Sour Cream

Regular	2 tablespoons	1 gram
Light	2 tablespoons	2 grams
Nonfat	2 tablespoons	4 grams

Cottage Cheese

Whole milk	½ cup	1.5 grams
2%	½ cup	4 grams
1%	½ cup	4 grams
Nonfat	½ cup	5 grams
Cream cheese	1 ounce	2 grams
Ricotta	½ cup	4 to 6 grams

Other Cheeses	1 ounce	under 1 gram

(American, Blue, Brie, Camembert, Cheddar, Colby, Edam, Farmer, Feta, Goat, Gouda, Gruyere, Havarti, Jarlsberg, Monterey Jack, Mozzarella, Muenster, Neufchâtel, Parmesan, Port du Salut, Provolone, Romano, Roquefort, String, Swiss.)

Ice Cream

Sugar-Free	½ cup	6–10 grams
Regular	½ cup	15 to 30 grams

Nuts, Seeds, Legumes

Almonds, dry-roasted	1 ounce	2 grams
Brazil nuts, dried	1 ounce	2 grams
Cashews, dry-roasted	1 ounce	7.5 grams
Cashews, honey-roasted	1 ounce	11 grams
Hazelnuts, dried	1 ounce	1.5 grams
Macadamia nuts, dried	1 ounce	1.5 grams
Peanuts, dry-roasted	1 ounce	4 grams
Peanut Butter	2 tablespoons	5 grams
Pistachio nuts, roasted	1 ounce	5.5 grams
Pumpkin seeds, dry-roasted	1 ounce	3 grams
Sunflower seeds, dry-roasted	1 ounce	3.5 grams
Walnuts, dried		
Black	1 ounce	3 grams
English	1 ounce	2 grams

Soy Products

Tofu	1 ounce	0.5 gram
Black soybeans	½ cup	4 grams
Miso	1 ounce	7.5 grams
Tempeh	1 ounce	1 gram
Soy milk, plain	1 cup	less than 1 gram

Resources

Low-Carb Tortillas:
  La Tortilla Factory
  Santa Rosa, CA
  (800)446-1516
  www.latortillafactory.com

Purveyors of natural grass-fed beef:
  Lasater Grasslands Beef
  (866)4LG-BEEF
  www.lasatergrasslandsbeef.com

Purveyors of wild game:
  New West Foods, Inc.
  1120 Lincoln Avenue Suite 905
  Denver, CO 80203
  (888)NEW-WEST
  www.NewWestFoods.com

Purveyor of fine cheese, crème
fraîche, and dairy products:
  Kendall Farms
  P.O. Box 686
  Atascadero, CA 93423
  (805) 466-7252

For more information about this diet or book, go to
www.30daylowcarbdietsolution.com.

Pertinent worthwhile reading on diet and exercise:

  The Low-Carb Comfort Food Cookbook, Mary Dan Eades, M.D., Michael R.
    Eades, M.D., and Ursula Solom (Wiley 2003).
  The Protein Power LifePlan, Michael R. Eades, M.D. and Mary Dan Eades,
    M.D. (Warner 2000).
  Protein Power, Michael R. Eades, M.D. and Mary Dan Eades, M.D. (Bantam
    1996).
  The Protein Power LifePlan Gram Counter, Michael R. Eades, M.D. and
    Mary Dan Eades, M.D. (Warner 2000).
  The Slow Burn Fitness Revolution, Michael R. Eades, M.D., Mary Dan
    Eades, M.D. and Frederick Hahn (Broadway 2003).
  The Paleo Diet, Loren Cordain, Ph.D. (Wiley 2002).
  The Good Fat Cookbook, Francis M. McCullough (Scribner 2003).

Newsletter:

  For a free sample issue of the *Eades Health Report* newsletter, write to
  Editor, Eades Health Report, P.O. Box 62, Denver, CO 80201 or click on
  www.eadeshealthreport.com, where you'll find up-to-date nutritional and
  health information.

Nutritional supplement information and dietary support:

  Also visit the Drs. Eades' site at *www.eatprotein.com* for information about
  available nutritional products, for dietary support, or to purchase books.

Meal Planner Worksheet

Protein Serving Size   _____ (S, M, L, XL, XXL)

Carbohydrate Serving Size   _____ (small, moderate, large)

	Yes	No
Did you take your multivitamin/mineral?	☐	☐
Did you take extra potassium/magnesium?	☐	☐

	What you planned to eat	What you actually ate
Breakfast:		
Protein serving	_____	_____
Carb serving	_____	_____
	_____	_____
Fluid (ounces)	_____	_____
Lunch:		
Protein serving	_____	_____
Carb serving	_____	_____
	_____	_____
Fluid (ounces)	_____	_____
Snack:	_____	_____
	_____	_____
Dinner:		
Protein serving	_____	_____
Carb serving	_____	_____
	_____	_____
Fluid (ounces)	_____	_____

Appendix B

Recommended Multivitamin and Mineral Profile

Vitamin/Mineral	Recommended Amount
Beta Carotene (for Vitamin A)	15,000 to 25,000 IU
Vitamin D_3[1]	50 to 100 IU
Ascorbic Acid (Vitamin C)	500 to 1000 mg
B Complex vitamins:	
Thiamine (Vitamin B_1)	100 mg
Riboflavin (Vitamin B_2)	40 mg
Niacin (Vitamin B_3)	110 mg
Pantothenic acid (Vitamin B_5)	400 to 500 mg
Pyridoxine (Vitamin B_6)	15 to 50 mg
Cobalamin (Vitamin B_{12})	250 to 800 *mcg*[2]
Folic Acid	800 mcg to 3 mg
Tocopherol (Vitamin E)	200 to 400 IU
Vitamin K_1	100 *mcg*
Boron	4 mg
Calcium (carbonate)	300 mg[3]
Magnesium (citrate, malate)	200 to 400 mg
Manganese (gluconate)	2 mg
Potassium (aspartate, gluconate)	99 mg–400 mg[4]
Vanadyl (sulfate)	100 *mcg*
Zinc (picolinate)	10 to 15 mg

[1] Supplement with vitamin D only if you eat no dietary sources (cod liver oil) and get no unblocked sun exposure on your skin.

[2] Abbreviation for micrograms—1/1000 of a milligram (mg).

[3] Assumes you eat regular dietary sources of calcium (dairy, especially). If not, increase to 1000 mg.

[4] It is not uncommon to experience a loss in potassium when you begin a low-carb diet as the body sheds excess fluid. We strongly recommend that you supplement with at least 200 mg of potassium daily in your first week or two on the program. Consult your pharmacist if you are taking medications for blood pressure or fluid retention prior to supplementing with extra potassium. Some of these medications cause you to retain potassium and your levels could become too high.

Appendix C

Visualizing Meat Portion Sizes

This page shows the approximate portion sizes for meat servings. It's useful to have a visual image of the size of your various protein and carbohydrate allotments.

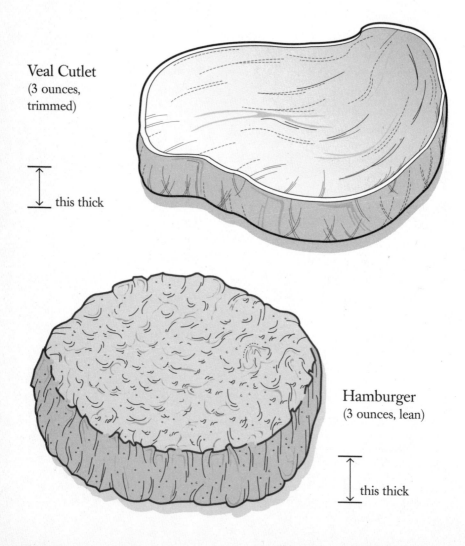

Veal Cutlet
(3 ounces, trimmed)

this thick

Hamburger
(3 ounces, lean)

this thick

Pork Chop
1 Chop (this size)
(3 ounces, fat removed)

this
thick

Roast Turkey
Roast Beef Round (lean only)
Ham (lean only)
3 ounces (2 slices
this size)

this
thick

Appendix D

Protein Requirements

Women

Weight	5' or less	5'1"	5'2"	5'3"	5'4"	5'5"	5'6"	5'7"	5'8"	5'9"	5'10"	5'11"	6' and up
up to 100	S	S	S	S	S	S	S	S	S	M	M	M	M
105	S	S	S	S	S	S	S	M	M	M	M	M	M
110	S	S	S	M	M	M	M	M	M	M	M	M	M
115	M	M	M	M	M	M	M	M	M	M	M	M	M
120	M	M	M	M	M	M	M	M	M	M	M	M	M
125	M	M	M	M	M	M	M	M	M	M	M	M	M
130	M	M	M	M	M	M	M	M	M	M	M	M	M
135	M	M	M	M	M	M	M	M	M	M	M	M	L
140	M	M	M	M	M	M	M	M	M	M	M	L	L
145	M	M	M	M	M	M	M	M	M	M	M	L	L
150	M	M	M	M	M	M	M	M	L	L	L	L	L
155	M	M	M	M	M	M	L	L	L	L	L	L	L
160	M	M	M	M	M	L	L	L	L	L	L	L	L
165	M	M	M	M	L	L	L	L	L	L	L	L	L
170	M	M	M	L	L	L	L	L	L	L	L	L	L
175	M	M	L	L	L	L	L	L	L	L	L	L	L
180	L	L	L	L	L	L	L	L	L	L	L	L	L
185	L	L	L	L	L	L	L	L	L	L	L	L	L
190	L	L	L	L	L	L	L	L	L	L	L	L	L
195	L	L	L	L	L	L	L	L	L	L	L	L	L
200	L	L	L	L	L	L	L	L	L	L	L	L	L
205	L	L	L	L	L	L	L	L	L	L	L	L	L
210	L	L	L	L	L	L	L	L	L	X	X	L	L
215	L	L	L	L	L	L	L	L	X	X	X	X	X
220	L	L	L	L	L	L	L	X	X	X	X	X	X
225	L	L	L	L	L	L	X	X	X	X	X	X	X
230	L	L	L	L	L	X	X	X	X	X	X	X	X
235	L	L	L	L	L	X	X	X	X	X	X	X	X
240	L	L	L	X	X	X	X	X	X	X	X	X	X
245	L	L	X	X	X	X	X	X	X	X	X	X	X
250	X	L	X	X	X	X	X	X	X	X	X	X	X
255	X	X	X	X	X	X	X	X	X	X	X	X	X
260	X	X	X	X	X	X	X	X	X	X	X	X	X
265	X	X	X	X	X	X	X	X	X	X	X	X	X
270	X	X	X	X	X	X	X	X	X	X	X	X	X
275	X	X	X	X	X	X	X	X	X	X	X	X	X
280	X	X	X	X	X	X	X	X	X	X	X	X	X
285	X	X	X	X	X	X	X	X	X	X	X	X	X
290	X	X	X	X	X	X	X	X	X	X	X	X	X
295	X	X	X	X	X	X	X	X	X	X	X	X	X
300 and up	X	X	X	X	X	X	X	X	X	X	X	X	X

Men

	Height															
Weight	5'4"	5'5"	5'6"	5'7"	5'8"	5'9"	5'10"	5'11"	6'0"	6'1"	6'2"	6'3"	6'4"	6'5"	6'6"	6'7" and up
up to 125	M	M	M	M	M	M	M	M	M	M	L	L	L	L	L	L
130	M	M	M	M	M	M	M	M	L	L	L	L	L	L	L	L
135	M	M	M	M	M	M	M	L	L	L	L	L	L	L	L	L
140	M	M	M	M	L	L	L	L	L	L	L	L	L	L	L	L
145	L	L	L	L	L	L	L	L	L	L	L	L	L	L	L	L
150	L	L	L	L	L	L	L	L	L	L	L	L	L	L	L	X
155	L	L	L	L	L	L	L	L	L	L	L	L	L	L	L	X
160	L	L	L	L	L	L	L	L	L	L	L	L	L	L	X	X
165	L	L	L	L	L	L	L	L	L	L	L	L	L	L	X	X
170	L	L	L	L	L	L	L	L	L	L	L	L	X	X	X	X
175	L	L	L	L	L	L	L	L	L	L	L	L	X	X	X	X
180	L	L	L	L	L	L	L	L	L	L	X	X	X	X	X	X
185	L	L	L	L	L	L	L	L	L	X	X	X	X	X	X	X
190	L	L	L	L	L	L	X	X	X	X	X	X	X	X	X	X
195	L	L	L	L	L	L	X	X	X	X	X	X	X	X	X	X
200	X	L	L	L	X	X	X	X	X	X	X	X	X	X	X	X
205	X	X	X	X	X	X	X	X	X	X	X	X	X	X	X	X
210	X	X	X	X	X	X	X	X	X	X	X	X	X	X	X	X
215	X	X	X	X	X	X	X	X	X	X	X	X	X	X	X	X
220	X	X	X	X	X	X	X	X	X	X	X	X	X	X	X	X
225	X	X	X	X	X	X	X	X	X	X	X	X	X	X	X	X
230	X	X	X	X	X	X	X	X	X	X	X	X	X	X	X	X
235	X	X	X	X	X	X	X	X	X	X	X	X	X	X	X	X
240	X	X	X	X	X	X	X	X	X	X	X	X	X	X	X	X
245	X	X	X	X	X	X	X	X	X	X	X	X	X	X	XX	XX
250	X	X	X	X	X	X	X	X	X	X	X	X	XX	XX	XX	XX
255	X	X	X	X	X	X	X	X	X	XX	XX	XX	XX	XX	XX	XX
260	X	X	X	X	X	X	XX	XX	XX	XX	XX	XX	XX	XX	XX	XX
265	X	X	X	X	XX	XX	XX	XX	XX	XX	XX	XX	XX	XX	XX	XX
270	X	X	XX	XX	XX	XX	XX	XX	XX	XX	XX	XX	XX	XX	XX	XX
275	X	XX	XX	XX	XX	XX	XX	XX	XX	XX	XX	XX	XX	XX	XX	XX
280	X	XX	XX	XX	XX	XX	XX	XX	XX	XX	XX	XX	XX	XX	XX	XX
285	XX	XX	XX	XX	XX	XX	XX	XX	XX	XX	XX	XX	XX	XX	XX	XX
290	XX	XX	XX	XX	XX	XX	XX	XX	XX	XX	XX	XX	XX	XX	XX	XX
295	XX	XX	XX	XX	XX	XX	XX	XX	XX	XX	XX	XX	XX	XX	XX	XX
300	XX	XX	XX	XX	XX	XX	XX	XX	XX	XX	XX	XX	XX	XX	XX	XX
305	XX	XX	XX	XX	XX	XX	XX	XX	XX	XX	XX	XX	XX	XX	XX	XX
310 and up	XX	XX	XX	XX	XX	XX	XX	XX	XX	XX	XX	XX	XX	XX	XX	XX

Index

alcohol, 40–41
almond extract, 154
almonds, 154
American Diabetic Association diet, 23
Anchovies, 111
anchovy fillets, 87
artificial sweeteners, 39
asparagus
    Asparagus Jayme, 122
    Asparagus Parmesano, 123
    Roast Pork Stir Fry, 100
aspartame, 39n
Avgolemono (Greek Egg-and-Lemon Soup), 92
avocado
    Sesame Tofu Salad, 90
    wraps, 95

bacon
    Casserole Egg-stravaganza, 74
    Kaye's Quiche, 76
    Sour Cream Beans, 127
bacon drippings
    Sour Cream Beans, 127
Baked Tofu Caesar Salad, 140
baking cocoa
    Hot Chocolate, 155
Barbecued Chicken Wings, 108
beef, barbecued
    wraps, 95
beef broth
    Homestyle Tomato Soup, 93
Beef K-Bobs, 97
beef tenderloin
    Easy Beef Tenderloin, 99

beer, 41
bell pepper. *See also* bell pepper entries below
    Beef K-Bobs, 97
    Breakfast Extravaganza, 73
    Shrimp K-Bobs, 121
    Skillet Ratatouille, 132
    Veggie Tofu Chili, 144
    Weight-Loss Chili, 98
bell pepper, green
    Salmon in Tomato Tubs, 118
bell pepper, red
    Skillet Chicken Italiano, 111
berries, mixed
    Mixed-Berry Syrup, 157
    Paleolithic Punch, 84
blackberries
    Mixed-Berry Syrup, 157
Blender Hollandaise Sauce, 165
blood sugar, regulating, 6–7, 23
blueberries
    Mixed-Berry Syrup, 157
Bravely Braised Cabbage, 134
bread crumbs, low-carb
    Sunday Spicy Chicken, 105
bread
    large serving list, 70
    medium serving list, 66
    small serving list, 63
breakfast
    Breakfast Burrito with Cream Cheese, 80
    Breakfast Extravaganza, 73
    Casserole Egg-stravaganza, 74
    Delightfully Devilish Eggs, 78
    Egg Salad, 77

Kaye's Quiche, 76
Lighter-than-Air Pancakes, 81
Paleolithic Punch, 84
Power Shake, 82
Sausage and Egg Breakfast Burrito, 79
Swiss Egg Casserole, 75
Veggie Frittata, 72
Yogurt Power Cup, 83
broccoli
Chicken Divan, 113
Salad de Floret, 89
Sautéed Broccoli, 124
Tofu and Broccoli Frittata, 147
Broiled Rosemary Veggie Burger, 143
brussels sprouts
Herbed Brussels Sprouts, 137
Buffalo mozzarella
Tomato and Mozzarella Salad, 85
Butter Lettuce Salad, 88

cabbage
Cabbage Lasagna, 145–46
Homemade Coleslaw, 86
Tangy Cabbage, 135
cabbage, green
Bravely Braised Cabbage, 134
Caesar dressing
Baked Tofu Caesar Salad, 140
Caesar Salad, 87
calories, 26, 38
capers
Delightfully Devilish Eggs, 78
Skillet Chicken Italiano, 111
carbohydrate contents, 169–70
carbohydrate restriction, medical conditions
treated with, 1
carbohydrates
adding, 32
controlling intake, 27–29
effect on insulin and glucagon, 12
identifying, 35–36
increasing intake, 57
carrots
Chef's Salad, 91
Hobo Dinner Pork Chops, 101
Homemade Coleslaw, 86
Casserole Egg-stravaganza, 74
cauliflower
Hobo Dinner Pork Chops, 101
Salad de Floret, 89
Zucchini Medley, 131
caviar
Delightfully Devilish Eggs, 78

cereal
large serving list, 70
medium serving list, 66
small serving list, 63
Charlie's Grilled Whole Fish, 119
cheese. *See also* cottage cheese, cream cheese,
other specific cheeses below
Kaye's Quiche, 76
wraps, 95
cheese, cheddar
Asparagus Parmesano, 123
Italian Zucchini Bake, 130
cheese, feta
Tofu and Broccoli Frittata, 147
cheese, hard
Chef's Salad, 91
Veggie Frittata, 72
cheese, monterey jack
Casserole Egg-stravaganza, 74
cheese, mozzarella
Cabbage Lasagna, 145–46
Tomato and Mozzarella Salad, 85 (Buffalo
mozzarella)
cheese, parmesan
Asparagus Parmesano, 123
Cabbage Lasagna, 145–46
Caesar Salad, 87
Chicken Divan, 113
Grilled Zucchini, 129
Roman-Style Chicken, 112
Salmon in Tomato Tubs, 118
Stuffed Veal, 102
Tofu and Broccoli Frittata, 147
Zucchini Medley, 131
cheese, ricotta
Cabbage Lasagna, 145–46
cheese, romano
Sassy Green Beans, 128
Zucchini Medley, 131
cheese, Roquefort
Roquefort Dressing, 159
cheese, swiss
Stuffed Veal, 102
Swiss Egg Casserole, 75
Chef's Salad, 91
chicken. *See also* chicken entries below
Cinder's Lemon Chicken, 106
Sunday Spicy Chicken, 105
Tabasco Chicken, 107
wraps, 95
chicken, barbecued
wraps, 95
chicken, canned
Chicken Salad, 114

chicken bouillon granules
    Chicken Divan, 113
chicken breast
    Chicken Divan, 113
    Roman-Style Chicken, 112
chicken breast, halves
    Grilled Chicken Breasts with Mustard, 110
    Rosemary Chicken, 109
chicken breast, skinned and boned
    Skillet Chicken Italiano, 111
chicken broth
    Asparagus Parmesano, 123
    Avgolemono (Greek Egg-and-Lemon
        Soup), 92
    Bravely Braised Cabbage, 134
    Sautéed Broccoli, 124
chicken salad
    Stuffed Tomato, 114
    wraps, 95
chicken stock
    Sadie Kendall's Mushroom Soup, 94
chicken thighs
    Roman-Style Chicken, 112
chicken wings
    Barbecued Chicken Wings, 108
Chocolate Butter Wafers, 153
chocolate chips, semi-sweet mini
    Mini Chocolate Chip Cheesecakes, 151
cholesterol
    lowering, 16–18
    low-fat diet ineffective for lowering, 18
chow mein vegetables
    Matilda's Marinated Green Beans, 125
Cinder's Lemon Chicken, 106
cocoa
    Chocolate Butter Wafers, 153
coconut, unsweetened
    Meringue Tart Shells, 154
condiments
    Blender Hollandaise Sauce, 165
    Crème Fraîche, 164
    Dry Rub for Meats, 166
    Homemade Mayonnaise, 163
    Italian Dressing, 160
    Minted Yogurt Dressing, 162
    Mr. Ron's Barbecue Sauce, 168
    Red Wine Vinaigrette, 158
    Roquefort Dressing, 159
    Tangy French Dressing, 161
    Versatile Meat Marinade, 167
cottage cheese
    Breakfast Burrito with Cream Cheese, 80
    Cabbage Lasagna, 145–46
    Lighter-than-Air Pancakes, 81
    Salad de Floret, 89

crab salad
    Stuffed Tomato, 114
cream cheese
    Breakfast Burrito with Cream Cheese, 80
    Delightfully Devilish Eggs, 78
    Lighter-than-Air Pancakes, 81
    Mini Chocolate Chip Cheesecakes, 151
    Strawberry Cheesecake, 150
cream of celery soup, concentrate
    Hobo Dinner Pork Chops, 101
Crème Fraîche, 164
    Chicken Divan, 113
    Sadie Kendall's Mushroom Soup, 94
cucumber
    Chef's Salad, 91
    Cukes and Onions, 136

dairy products, carbohydrate contents, 169–70
deli meats
    wraps, 95
Delightfully Devilish Eggs, 78
desserts
    Chocolate Butter Wafers, 153
    Hot Chocolate, 155
    Meringue Tart Shells, 154
    Mini Chocolate Chip Cheesecakes, 151
    Orange and Strawberry Cup, 149
    Simple Nut Crust for   152
    Strawberry Cheesecake, 150
diabetes, 3, 23
Dia-Mel Diet Catsup
    Mr. Ron's Barbecue Sauce, 168
dietary fat, 10
diets, assessing, 4–5
dill pickle
    Egg Salad, 77
    Chicken Salad, 114
dill pickle relish
    Veggie-Stuffed Avocado (Tofu and Egg
        Salad), 142
    wraps, 95
distilled spirits, 41
Dry Rub for Meats, 166

Easy Beef Tenderloin, 99
Easy Pork Tenderloin, 99
effective carbohydrate content, 32n
egg dishes
    Breakfast Extravaganza, 73
    Casserole Egg-stravaganza, 74
    Delightfully Devilish Eggs, 78
    Egg Salad, 77
    Kaye's Quiche, 76
    Sausage and Egg Breakfast Burrito, 79
    Swiss Egg Casserole, 75
    Veggie Frittata, 72

eggplant
 Breakfast Extravaganza, 73
 Eggplant Milano, 133
 Skillet Ratatouille, 132
Egg Salad, 77
 wraps, 95
exercise, 19
extra-extra-large serving list, protein, 60
extra-large serving list, protein, 59

Fancy Green Beans, 126
fats, 29–30, 37–38
Featherweight Diet Catsup, Mr. Ron's Barbecue
 Sauce, 168
fiber, 11–12
fish
 wraps, 95
fish, whole
 Charlie's Grilled Whole Fish, 119
fish dishes
 Charlie's Grilled Whole Fish, 119
 Fish and Peppers, 116
 Grilled Salmon Steaks with Chive Butter,
 117
 Halibut Jardinere, 115
 Salmon in Tomato Tubs, 118
 Shrimp K-Bobs, 121
 Skillet Shrimp, 120
 Tuna Salad, 114
flounder fillets
 Fish and Peppers, 116
Lighter-than-Air Pancakes, 81
fluid retention, 7
fluids, 38–39
food, key to metabolic balance, 9–10
fructose, 11
fruit, 36. See also blackberries, blueberries,
 orange, strawberries
 large serving list, 67–68
 medium serving list, 64
 Meringue Tart Shells, 154
 small serving list, 61

glucagon, 6, 12
glucose, 11, 15
"good" HDL cholesterol, raising, 18–19
grains
 large serving list, 70
 medium serving list, 66
 small serving list, 63
green beans. See also green bean entries below
 Fancy Green Beans, 126
 Sassy Green Beans, 128

green beans, french-cut
 Matilda's Marinated Green Beans, 125
 Sour Cream Beans, 127
green beans, Italian
 Skillet Chicken Italiano, 111
Grilled Chicken Breasts with Mustard, 110
Grilled Lamb Burgers, 96
Grilled Salmon Steaks with Chive Butter, 117
Grilled Zucchini, 129
ground beef
 Weight-Loss Chili, 98
guar gum
 Mixed-Berry Syrup, 157

Halibut Jardinère, 115
ham
 Chef's Salad, 91
ham, boiled
 Stuffed Veal, 102
hamburger
 wraps, 95
heart disease, 3–4
 elevated triglycerides linked to, 18
 reducing risk, 19–20
hen, roasting
 Roasted Paprika Chicken, 104
Herbed Brussels Sprouts, 137
high blood pressure, 7
Hobo Dinner Pork Chops, 101
Homemade Coleslaw, 86
Homemade Mayonnaise, 163
 Homemade Coleslaw, 86
 Tangy Cabbage, 135
 Veggie Pita TLT, 141
 Veggie-Stuffed Avocado (Tofu and Egg
 Salad), 142
 wraps, 95
Homestyle Tomato Soup, 93
hormones, 10
Hot Chocolate, 155
hyperinsulinemia, 6

insulin, 6
 effect of carbohydrates on, 12
 effect on heart disease, 19
 lowering levels of, 8
 relation to diseases, 1, 4
insulin receptors, 6–7
insulin-related health problems, inventory for,
 8–9
insulin resistance, 7, 17
Italian Dressing, 160
Italian Zucchini Bake, 130

Kaye's Quiche, 76
ketones, 39

lamb
　　Grilled Lamb Burgers, 96
　　wraps, 95
large serving lists
　　carbohydrate, 66–70
　　protein, 59
lean body mass, preserving 20–22
legumes, carbohydrate contents, 170
lemons
　　Avgolemono (Greek Egg-and-Lemon
　　　　Soup), 92
　　Cinder's Lemon Chicken, 106
lettuce. *See also* lettuce entries below
　　wraps, 95
lettuce, butter
　　Butter Lettuce Salad, 88
lettuce, iceberg
　　Chef's Salad, 91
lettuce, large leaf
　　Veggie Pita TLT, 141
lettuce, loose leaf
　　Chef's Salad, 91
lettuce, mixed
　　Sesame Tofu Salad, 90
lettuce, romaine
　　Baked Tofu Caesar Salad, 140
　　Caesar Salad, 87
liver, function of, 18
livestock, fattening diet of, 14
Low-Carb Comfort Food Cookbook (Eades &
　　Eades), 34, 43
low-carb diets
　　calories and, 26
　　criticism of, 15
　　eating by color, 33–34
　　effects of, 10, 24
　　fat intake on, 29–30
　　foods to eat and foods to avoid, 33–34,
　　　　36–43
　　graduating to more carbs, 32
　　meal planning for, 31
　　medications and, 17n, 23, 29
　　protein requirements, 25–26, 35
　　protein's importance to, 27
　　rules for, 24, 31
　　30-day expectations, 30–31
low-carb lifestyle, health benefits of
　　controlling blood sugar, 23
　　lowering cholesterol and triglycerides,
　　　　16–18
　　preserving lean body, 20–22
　　raising "good" HDL cholesterol, 18–19
　　reduced heart disease risk, 19–20

Low-Carb Pyramid, 16
low-fat diets, effects of, 3, 8

Mango Smoothie, 148
Matilda's Marinated Green Beans, 125
meal intervals, 27
meal planning, 31, 44
　　carbohydrate serving lists, 60–70
　　generic, 45
　　protein serving lists, 58–60
　　substitutions in, 42–43
　　30-day meal planner, 45–57
　　worksheet, 172
meat dishes
　　Beef K-Bobs, 97
　　Easy Beef Tenderloin, 99
　　Easy Pork Tenderloin, 99
　　Grilled Lamb Burgers, 96
　　Hobo Dinner Pork Chops, 101
　　Roast Pork Stir Fry, 100
　　Stuffed Veal, 102
　　Venison Tenderloin with Rosemary Sauce,
　　　　103
　　Weight-Loss Chili, 98
meats, portion sizes, 174–75
medium serving lists
　　carbohydrate, 63–66
　　protein, 58
Meringue Tart Shells, 154
metabolic balance, 6, 9–10
metabolic rate
　　food's effect on, 12–13
　　protein intake related to, 27
minerals, recommended, 173
mineral supplements, 40
Mini Chocolate Chip Cheesecakes, 151
Minted Yogurt Dressing, 162
　　wraps, 95
Mixed-Berry Syrup, 157
Mr. Ron's Barbecue Sauce, 168
　　wraps, 95
Muir Glen Organic regular catsup
　　Mr. Ron's Barbecue Sauce, 168
multivitamins, recommended, 173
mushrooms
　　Beef K-Bobs, 97
　　Breakfast Extravaganza, 73
　　Halibut Jardinère, 115
　　Matilda's Marinated Green Beans, 125
　　Roast Pork Stir Fry, 100
　　Roman-Style Chicken, 112
　　Sadie Kendall's Mushroom Soup, 94
　　Shrimp K-Bobs, 121
　　Stewart's Mushrooms, 139
　　Veggie Frittata, 72

Veggie Tofu Chili, 144
Weight-Loss Chili, 98
mushrooms, white
Sautéed Mushrooms, 138

nutritional knowledge, test of, 5–6
nutritional supplements, 40
nuts, carbohydrate contents, 170

obesity, rise in, 3
oils, 29–30, 38
olive oil Italian dressing
Skillet Shrimp, 120
olives, black
Delightfully Devilish Eggs, 78
Egg Salad, 77
onion. *See also* onion entries below
Beef K-Bobs, 97
Cabbage Lasagna, 145–46
Cinder's Lemon Chicken, 106
Egg Salad, 77
Eggplant Milano, 133
green, Chef's Salad, 91
Grilled Chicken Breasts with Mustard, 110
Grilled Lamb Burgers, 96
Halibut Jardinère, 115
Herbed Brussels Sprouts, 137
Hobo Dinner Pork Chops, 101
Kaye's Quiche, 76
Roasted Paprika Chicken, 104
Roast Pork Stir Fry, 100
Roman-Style Chicken, 112
Sadie Kendall's Mushroom Soup, 94
Sassy Green Beans, 128
Shrimp K-Bobs, 121
Veggie Tofu Chili, 144
Weight-Loss Chili, 98
onion, green
Salmon in Tomato Tubs, 118
onion, white
Breakfast Extravaganza, 73
Cukes and Onions, 136
Mr. Ron's Barbecue Sauce, 168
Skillet Ratatouille, 132
onion, yellow
Charlie's Grilled Whole Fish, 119
orange, mandarin
Butter Lettuce Salad, 88
orange, valencia
Orange and Strawberry Cup, 149
Ornish, Dean, 20

Paleolithic Punch, 84
pecans
Mini Chocolate Chip Cheesecakes, 151

Simple Nut Crust for Desserts, 152
Yogurt Power Cup, 83
pepper, green
Halibut Jardinere, 115
pepper, green chili
Fish and Peppers, 116
pepper, red, roasted
Tofu and Broccoli Frittata, 147
peppers. *See* bell pepper
Pickapeppa Sauce
Stewart's Mushrooms, 139
pimiento
Halibut Jardinere, 115
Matilda's Marinated Green Beans, 125
Skillet Chicken Italiano, 111
pineapple juice, unsweetened
Roast Pork Stir Fry, 100
pork, barbecued
wraps, 95
pork, roasted
Roast Pork Stir Fry, 100
pork chops
Hobo Dinner Pork Chops, 101
pork tenderloin
Easy Pork Tenderloin, 99
portion sizes, 25, 26
Power Shake, 82
preserves
Strawberry Preserves, 156
protein, 10
distributing intake, 26
importance of, 27
requirements, 25–26, 35
role in self-preservation, 21
serving lists, 58–60
serving sizes, 176–77
protein powder
Mango Smoothie, 148
Power Shake, 82
Protein Power (Eades & Eades), 1, 2, 20
The Protein Power LifePlan (Eades & Eades),
1, 2

raspberries
Mixed-Berry Syrup, 157
red snapper, whole
Charlie's Grilled Whole Fish, 119
Red Wine Vinaigrette, 158
rice flour
Lighter-than-Air Pancakes, 81
Roast Pork Stir Fry, 100
Roasted Paprika Chicken, 104
Roman-Style Chicken, 112
Roquefort Dressing, 159
Rosemary Chicken, 109

Sadie Kendall's Mushroom Soup, 94
Salad de Floret, 89
salads
    Butter Lettuce Salad, 88
    Caesar Salad, 87
    Chef's Salad, 91
    Homemade Coleslaw, 86
    Salad de Floret, 89
    Sesame Tofu Salad, 90
    Tomato and Mozzarella Salad, 85
salmon
    Delightfully Devilish Eggs, 78
salmon, canned pink
    Salmon in Tomato Tubs, 118
salmon steaks
    Grilled Salmon Steaks with Chive Butter,
        117
salsa
    Sausage and Egg Breakfast Burrito, 79
Sassy Green Beans, 128
Sausage and Egg Breakfast Burrito, 79
Sautéed Broccoli, 124
Sautéed Mushrooms, 138
seeds, carbohydrate contents, 170
Sesame Tofu Salad, 90
shallots
    Grilled Chicken Breasts with Mustard, 110
    Homestyle Tomato Soup, 93
    Sadie Kendall's Mushroom Soup, 94
shrimp, medium
    Skillet Shrimp, 120
shrimp, large
    Shrimp K-Bobs, 121
shrimp salad
    Stuffed Tomato, 114
    wraps, 95
Simple Nut Crust for Desserts, 152
Skillet Chicken Italiano, 111
Skillet Ratatouille, 132
Skillet Shrimp, 120
small serving lists
    carbohydrate, 60–63
    protein, 58
snacks, 41–42
SoBe Lean, Power Shake, 82
sole fillets
    Fish and Peppers, 116
soups
    Avgolemono (Greek Egg-and-Lemon
        Soup), 92
    Homestyle Tomato Soup, 93
    Sadie Kendall's Mushroom Soup, 94
Sour Cream Beans, 127
soy milk, unsweetened
    Mango Smoothie, 148

soy products, carbohydrate contents, 170
spinach
    Kaye's Quiche, 76
    Veggie Frittata, 72
sprouts
    Veggie Pita TLT, 141
starches, 11, 37
steak
    wraps, 95
steak cubes
    Beef K-Bobs, 97
Stewart's Mushrooms, 139
strawberries
    Breakfast Burrito with Cream Cheese, 80
    Mixed-Berry Syrup, 157
    Orange and Strawberry Cup, 149
    Strawberry Cheesecake, 150
    Strawberry Preserves, 156
stroke, 3–4
Stuffed Tomato, 114
Stuffed Veal, 102
substitutions, 42–43
sugars, 11
Sunday Spicy Chicken, 105
sweeteners, 39
Swiss Egg Casserole, 75
syrup
    Mixed-Berry Syrup, 157

Tabasco Chicken, 107
Tangy Cabbage, 135
Tangy French Dressing, 161
Taubes, Gary, 1–2
Thin So Fast (Eades & Eades), 1
tofu, baked
    wraps, 95
tofu, pre-baked, pre-seasoned
    Baked Tofu Caesar Salad, 140
tofu, pre-cooked
    Veggie-Stuffed Avocado (Tofu and Egg
        Salad), 142
tofu, pre-seasoned
    Veggie Pita TLT, 141
Tofu and Broccoli Frittata, 147
tomato
    Chef's Salad, 91
    Chicken Salad, 114
    Eggplant Milano, 133
    Halibut Jardinere, 115
    Homestyle Tomato Soup, 93
    Italian Zucchini Bake, 130
    Roast Pork Stir Fry, 100
    Roman-Style Chicken, 112
    Salmon in Tomato Tubs, 118
    Skillet Chicken Italiano, 111

Skillet Ratatouille, 132
Tomato and Mozzarella Salad, 85
Tuna Salad, 114
Veggie Pita TLT, 141
Veggie Tofu Chili, 144
Weight-Loss Chili, 98
wraps, 95
Zucchini Medley, 131
tomato juice
Sassy Green Beans, 128
Tomato and Mozzarella Salad, 85
tortilla, low-carb
Breakfast Burrito with Cream Cheese, 80
ordering information, 171
Sausage and Egg Breakfast Burrito, 79
wraps, 95
trans fats, 30
triglycerides, lowering, 16–18
trout, whole
Charlie's Grilled Whole Fish, 119
Tuna Salad, 114
Stuffed Tomato, 114
wraps, 95
type II diabetes, 3, 23

ultra-low-carb diet, 17
USDA food pyramid, 12–14

veal cutlets
Stuffed Veal, 102
vegetable dishes
Asparagus Jayme, 122
Asparagus Parmesano, 123
Bravely Braised Cabbage, 134
Cukes and Onions, 136
Eggplant Milano, 133
Fancy Green Beans, 126
Grilled Zucchini, 129
Herbed Brussels Sprouts, 137
Italian Zucchini Bake, 130
Matilda's Marinated Green Beans, 125
Sassy Green Beans, 128
Sautéed Broccoli, 124
Sautéed Mushrooms, 138
Skillet Ratatouille, 132
Sour Cream Beans, 127
Stewart's Mushrooms, 139
Tangy Cabbage, 135
Zucchini Medley, 131
vegetable protein hamburger substitute
Cabbage Lasagna, 145–46
Veggie Tofu Chili, 144
vegetables, 36–37
large serving list, 68–69
medium serving list, 64–66
small serving list, 61–62

vegetarian dishes
Baked Tofu Caesar Salad, 140
Broiled Rosemary Veggie Burger, 143
Cabbage Lasagna, 145–46
Mango Smoothie, 148
Tofu and Broccoli Frittata, 147
Veggie Pita TLT, 141
Veggie-Stuffed Avocado (Tofu and Egg
Salad), 142
Veggie Tofu Chili, 144
veggie burgers
Broiled Rosemary Veggie Burger, 143
wraps, 95
Veggie Frittata, 72
Veggie Pita TLT, 141
Veggie-Stuffed Avocado (Tofu and Egg Salad),
142
Veggie Tofu Chili, 144
Venison Tenderloin with Rosemary Sauce, 103
Versatile Meat Marinade, 167
vitamins, 40

walnuts
Butter Lettuce Salad, 88
Simple Nut Crust for Desserts, 152
water, 38–39
water chestnuts
Fancy Green Beans, 126
Matilda's Marinated Green Beans, 125
Weight-Loss Chili, 98
What If Fat Doesn't Make You Fat? (Taubes),
1–2
wine, 40–41
wine (dry, red or white)
Sautéed Mushrooms, 138
wine, dry white
Stuffed Veal, 102
wine, white
Halibut Jardinère, 115
wraps, 95

yogurt, plain
Yogurt Power Cup, 83
yogurt, unsweetened
Minted Yogurt Dressing, 162
Yogurt Power Cup, 83

zucchini
Grilled Zucchini, 129
Italian Zucchini Bake, 130
Skillet Ratatouille, 132
Zucchini Medley, 131
zucchini squash
Hobo Dinner Pork Chops, 101
Roman-Style Chicken, 112

The
Low-Carb Comfort Food
Cookbook

By Michael R. Eades, M.D.,
Mary Dan Eades, M.D.,
and Ursula Solom

More than 300 recipes that will satisfy your comfort-food
cravings while keeping you thin

Join the
30-Day Low-Carb Diet Solution Challenge

Lose weight—Win prizes

www.30daylowcarbdietsolution.com